HEMORRHOIDS: SYMPTOMS, DIAGNOSIS AND TREATMENT

HEMORRHOIDS: SYMPTOMS, DIAGNOSIS AND TREATMENT

PHILIP D. SALINITRI
AND
BENJAMIN M. RASPALLO
EDITORS

Nova Science Publishers, Inc.
New York

For permission to use material from this book please contact us:
Telephone 631-231-7269; Fax 631-231-8175
Web Site: http://www.novapublishers.com

Library of Congress Cataloging-in-Publication Data

Hemorrhoids : symptoms, diagnosis, and treatment / editors, Philip D. Salinitri and Benjamin M. Raspallo.
p. ; cm.
Includes bibliographical references and index.
ISBN 978-1-60876-478-5 (hardcover : alk. paper)
1. Hemorrhoids. I. Salinitri, Philip D. II. Raspallo, Benjamin M.
[DNLM: 1. Hemorrhoids. WI 605 H489 2009]
RC865.H46 2009
616.3'52--dc22

2009040470

Published by Nova Science Publishers, Inc. † New York

Contents

PREFACE

Hemorrhoidal disease is the consequence of pathological changes of fibrovascular anal cushions producing symptoms. Symptomatic hemorrhoids may include bleeding, prolapse, pruritus, soiling, thrombosis and pain. Different invasive treatment modalities are explored, which vary from office treatment (rubber bands, sclerotherapy, infrared coagulation, cryotherapy) and surgical procedure (hemorrhoidectomy, stapled hemorrhoidopexy). Only 5-10% of patients require surgery. The authors of this book review and discuss recent innovations of post-hemorrhoidectomy pain control and wound healing. Stapled haemorrhoidopexy (SH) as an attractive alternative to conventional haemorrhoidectomy (CH) is looked at as well. In addition, new techniques (Doppler guided transanal haemorrhoidal dearterialisation) with new devices in order to attain improved patient satisfaction (THD and haemorrhoid laser procedure) is analyzed. Finally, anal ultra slow wave (USW), a manometric finding observed in some patients with hemorrhoids, is presented and its clinical relevance is discussed.

Chapter 1 – Hemorrhoidal disease is the consequence of pathological changes of fibrovascular anal cushions producing symptoms. Symptomatic hemorrhoids may present with bleeding, prolapse, pruritus, soiling, thrombosis and pain. All the potential differential diagnoses of hemorrhoidal disease must be considered in the diagnostic process, as many different colorectal diseases may cause overlapping signs and symptoms.

Treatment includes conservative management (dietary management and lifestyle modifications), which may be effective in the treatment of grade I and some grade II hemorrhoids. Patients still reporting symptoms after conservative management may be candidates for minimally invasive office procedures. These are recommended for most patients with refractory grade I, grade II or grade III hemorrhoids. Surgical hemorrhoidectomy is the treatment of choice for grade IV hemorrhoids, strangulated hemorrhoids and some symptomatic grade III hemorrhoids. Surgical excision is also indicated when minimally invasive office procedures fail to relieve hemorrhoidal symptoms and when patients are not able to tolerate office procedures. Only 5-10% of patients require surgery. Surgical hemorrhoidectomy is considered the most effective treatment for hemorrhoids with fewer recurrences. However, it is associated with more pain and postoperative disability compared to minimally invasive office procedures.

Chapter 2 - Hemorrhoids are one of the most frequent pathologies, with an estimated prevalence of 4.4%. Treatment strategies are various and can be divided into conservative therapies (either paharmacological or instrumental) and surgery.

Medical therapy includes vasoactive agents (flavonoids) and various topical agents aiming to reduce symptoms.

Instrumental therapies (elastic band ligation, sclerotherapy, cryotherapy, cauterization, etc.) can be effective in about 70–90% of patients in the short term with a significant rate of recurrence in the long term.

Surgical therapy guaranties satisfactory results, which are significantly better that those obtained with conservative therapies, especially for grade III and IV hemorrhoids. Traditional surgery for hemorrhoids aims to remove the hemorroids, with closure (Fergusson's technique) or without closure (Milligan-Morgan procedure) of the ensuing defect. This traditional approach is effective, but causes significant postoperative pain because of wide external wounds in the innervated perianal skin. Stapled hemorrhopidopexy, proposed by Longo, has gained vast acceptance because of less postoperative pain and faster return to normal activities. This technique aims to reduce the hemorrhoidal prolapse by repositioning the hemorrhoidal masses into the anal canal and by reducing the venous engorgement with transaction of feeding arteries and redundant mucosa. The procedure results in a stapled mucosa anastomosis in the rectum, at least 3 cm above the dentate line where sensitive receptors are few, without any dissection or trauma in the area of anal mucosa and anoderm.

The superiority of stapled hemorrhoidopexy in terms of less postoperative pain and quicker recovery was confirmed by a recent systematic review of 25 randomized trials comparing stapled hemorrhoidopexy and conventional hemorrhoidectomy. However, the long-term control of hemorrhoid symptoms as well as the recurrence of prolapsing hemorrhoids should be addressed in order to draw a final conclusion about the efficacy and effectiveness of stapled hemorrhoidopexy. In the recent literature, a significant incidence of recurrence after stapled hemorrhoidopexy was reported. In particular, when compared with conventional hemorrhoidectomy, stapled hemorrhoidopexy resulted in a higher incidence of recurrence and a worse clinical outcome. The higher recurrence rate may be sometimes the result of inappropriate patient selection. Therefore, with the presence of large-volume prolapsing internal hemorrhoids, we could imagine that stapled hemorrhoidopexy using two staplers would not be appropriate. Further prospective studies with more attention to appropriate patient selection are necessary to assess the efficacy of the various surgical procedures for hemorrhoids.

Chapter 3 - Stapled haemorrhoidopexy (SH) is an attractive alternative to conventional haemorrhoidectomy (CH) because of reduced postoperative pain, shorter hospital stay and earlier return to normal activities. Over the last decade, SH gained wide acceptance but this enthusiastic use has been tempered by increasing reports of specific technique related complications including occasional life threatening sepsis and deaths. Complications rate has been reported as high as 31%.

Data on patients undergoing haemorrhoidectomy at our unit or referred to us are prospectively entered in a database.

Patients and methods: We report our experience on 425 symptomatic patients who underwent haemorrhoidectomy at our Institution: 110 underwent SH while 315 underwent conventional haemorrhoidectomy with similar follow-up period (25±14 vs 32±16 months).

Clinical outcome was assessed by a validated questionnaire on postoperative symptoms and satisfaction supplemented by the Wexner incontinence score. Data on bleeding, body temperature, pain after defecation, prolapse, incontinence, faecal urgency was prospectively recorded and analysed using Fisher exact and Mann-Whitney tests.

Results: Operating time between SH and CH was similar being 28.3±8.7 and 26±8.8 minutes respectively. Hospitalization rates were similar between SH and CH (2.7% vs 1.6%).

Likewise, no differences were observed in terms of ER admissions (7.3% vs 3.8%) and hospital readmissions (3.6% vs 2.2%) between SH and CH.

Overall early and late complication rates were similar between SH and CH.

Despite an increased quote of anal fissure, disabling chronic pain and recurrences were observed after SH when compared to CH, no significative differences were observed in terms of early and late complications between SH and CH (please refer to tables I and II).

Significant differences were observed in terms of pain (expressed as VAS) during the first postoperative week (please refer to figures 1 and 2). Patients who underwent CH experienced more severe pain (expressed as VAS score >7) than SH at 5, 6 and 7 postoperative day. We did not observed differences between SH and CH in terms of postoperative pain and severe pain (VAS >7) among third and fourth degree haemorrhoids.

Postoperative symptoms duration including pain, bleeding, soiling and hitching lasted more after CH compared to SH reaching significant differences for soiling and bleeding (please refer to figure 3).

Postoperative fever was similar between the two groups. No differences were observed in terms of return to work expressed in days between the SH and CH.

Urgency after 3 months was significantly more frequent after SH compared to CH (8.2% vs 0.6%), despite this difference disappeared at 1 year (0.9% vs 0.3%).

Three patients (2.7%) experienced severe disabling chronic pain after SH that lasted >1 year since surgery without the expected improvement over the follow-up. Early haemorrhoidal recurrences (as thrombosis) occurred 4 and 12 days after surgery. Six patients developed late haemorrhoidal recurrence after 16±5 months from previous surgery. Twelve patients experienced transient urgency (10.9%) that resolved within 4 months in all patients but one in which lasted 13 months. Two patients (1.8%) developed symptomatic rectal stricture with urgency and frequency and responded to anal dilatation with anal dilators. Overall reinterventions rate after SH was 9.1% (vs 4.8% of CH, not significant).

Chapter 4 - Hemorrhoidopathy is a common disease in the western world. It is believed that 20-30% of all people will develop symptomatic hemorrhoids at a stage of their life. It is one of the commonest benign pathologies that surgeons treat on their daily medical practice. Therefore, a large number of options have been developed for the treatment of hemorrhoids, each of them having certain indications and applications.

Hemorrhoids are normal anatomical formations of the human anal canal, playing an important role in the closure mechanism of the anal ring. The pathogenesis of hemorrhoidopathy is still not completely known, and many theories on its development have been published and debated upon. Hemorrhoids are divided in 4 stages, depending on the degree of prolapse and need for reduction. Stage 1 and 2 hemorrhoids are usually managed conservatively, whereas hemorrhoids of stage 3 and 4 often have to be treated surgically.

In 1998, Antonio Longo suggested the reduction of hemorrhoids and fixation of the prolapsing mucosa for the treatment of hemorrhoids in a technique known as PPH (Procedure for Prolapse and Hemorrhoids). When performing a PPH, a circular segment of mucosa and submucosa of the rectum is resected 2 centimeters proximal to the dentate line, using a circular stapler. For the resection, a purse-string suture is applied and tied at the 3 o'clock position. In our department, we modify the technique by applying a second suture at the 9 o'clock position. This allows us to provide a symmetrical retraction of the mucosa and submucosa into the stapler. The circular resection fixes the prolapsing mucosa and reduces the hemorrhoids. Furthermore, the staple line ligates the end branches of the superior haemorrhoidal artery, an action which reduces the blood supply to the hemorrhoids.

The procedure can be performed under general or spinal anesthesia and there is no need for prolonged hospital stay for the patient. The main advantage of the hemorrhoidopexy is the absence of postoperative pain, which was the main problem following a classical Milligan-Morgan hemorrhoidectomy. The main complications of the hemorrhoidopexy are urgency, hemorrhage and stenosis of the anal canal. The frequency of complications after PPH ranges between 6% and 31%.

In the last 10 years we performed hemorrhoidopexy in 812 patients in our department. All operations were performed under general anesthesia. The mean operating time was 14.3 minutes and the mean hospital stay 1.1 days. Postoperatively, 28 patients (3.4%) complained of mild pain for 2-9 days which was treated with plain oral analgesics. Three patients (0.3%) developed postoperative bleeding, 2 of them were treated conservatively and 1 had to be re-operated for haemostasis.

In conclusion, hemorrhoidopexy is a simple, effective, pain-free method for the treatment of mainly 3rd degree hemorrhoids with many advantages compared to the conventional hemorrhoidectomy.

Chapter 5 – Introduction: The lower cost of the procedure associated with a good long term cosmetic effect in patients with large skin tags make open excision hemorrhoidectomy a viable option still.

It is not uncommon however for surgical excision of hemorrhoids to be associated with postoperative pain together with perianal discharge, itchiness and irritation during the healing phase. Some recent local studies have provided us some insight into improving wound healing rates and postoperative pain after excision hemorrhoidectomy. This article reviews and discusses recent innovations of post-hemorrhoidectomy pain control and wound healing.

Improving Outcome after Excision Hemorrhoidectomy: There is no doubt that postoperative spasm of the internal sphincter contributes to pain and poor wound healing. Topical glyceryl trinitrate (GTN) reduces anal canal pressures and improves anodermal blood flow. Post-hemorrhoidectomy topical use of GTN may reduce anal spasm and improve postoperative pain while improved anodermal blood flow may accelerate wound healing.

In another local study looking at the addition of methylene blue to local analgesics to prolong postoperative local anesthetic effect, we found that methylene blue was effective in prolonging anesthesia for up to about 3 weeks.

More recently, several randomized trials comparing diathermy haemorrhoidectomy to Ligasure hemorrhoidectomy have also found improvement in pain and healing using Ligasure. Dissection with Ligasure is associated with a reduced collateral damage to adjacent tissue compared to diathermy. The reduced anal spasm and smaller open wounds associated with Ligasure hemorrhoidectomy may have contributed to earlier wound healing.

Conclusion: Recent studies have provided some new methods for improving the postoperative outcomes of the technique of excision hemorrhoidectomy. Wound healing rates may be improved by topical glyceryl trinitrate which improves anodermal blood flow and also with the usage of Ligasure. The addition of methylene blue for topical analgesics may allow a prolongation of analgesic which may allow for a more painless recovery. More studies are currently being conducted for further improvement of results in an operation that is frequently indicated in our population.

Chapter 6 - Stapled hemorrhoidopexy is increasingly practiced in treatment of hemorrhoidal disease. For an ideal application of this method, purse-string suture must be put at a certain distance with appropriate thickness. This may sometimes be difficult, and an unsuitable purse string suture placement may increase the risk of postoperative complications. The videoanoscope was created to prevent the difficulties during application of the purse-string suture.

The videoanoscope consists of three pieces: the front piece with an open top gradually narrows and makes a nozzle at the tip; the top piece is a sliding lid that covers the front piece; and the back piece has a handle that allows insertion of a 10 mm telescope in order to shed light inside the anoscope and transfer images to the monitor.

The sliding lid forms a window above the anoscope when pulled back, and allows suturing rectal mucosa that hangs down into the anoscope. Suturing may be continued by rotating the anoscope clockwise direction, and it is completed upon reaching the start point.

The purse-string suture placement and the stapled haemorrhoidopexy procedure were easily performed by using the videoanoscope. Additionally, it is possible to get the view inside of the anoscope, and the procedure can be viewed on a monitor. Moreover it has some advantages such as recording the operation by videoanoscope, and these records may be useful for surgical training.

Chapter 7 - Hemorrhoidal disease is a common problem in the western world (in USA, ten million, just < 5 percent of the population ([1]).

Different invasive treatment modalities are available for the management of the symptomatic haemorrhoids varying from office treatment (rubber bands, sclerotherapy ,infrared coagulation, cryotherapy) and surgical procedure (hemorrhoidectomy, stapled hemorrhoidopexy)

The high frequency of this entity and the deterioration in quality of life during the initial postoperative period has led the implementation of new technique (Doppler guided transanal haemorrhoidal dearterialisation) with new devices in order to attain improved patient satisfaction (THD and haemorrhoid laser procedure).

Chapter 8 - Anal ultra slow wave (USW) is a manometric finding observed in some patients with hemorrhoids and is assumed to represent a hyperactive internal anal sphincter. Lateral sphincterotomy has been reported as a treatment option in patients with hemorrhoids exhibiting USW to reduce the activity of the internal anal sphincter. Hemorrhoids in the anal canal were once thought to induce USW; however, the underlining mechanism of USW is not known. Hyperactivity of the internal anal sphincter, namely hypertonic anal canal, may cause difficulty in defecation. In fact, USW is also observed in some patients without hemorrhoids but with megacolon, chronic constipation, spina bifida, and anal fissure. We found USW in four out of 70 children with chronic constipation. The origin of USW is thought to be the internal anal sphincter because some patients with spina bifida with a completely flaccid external anal sphincter can exhibit USW. The natural history of patients with USW is not known. In some cases, histological change in intestinal ganglion cells is observed. In this commentary, USW is presented and its clinical relevance is discussed with a special interest to the manometric findings of hemorrhoids.

In: Hemorrhoids: Symptoms, Diagnosis… ISBN: 978-1-60876-478-5
Authors: P. Salinitri et al., pp. 1-23

Chapter 1

HEMORRHOIDS: SYMPTOMS, DIAGNOSIS AND TREATMENTS

Francesco Di Fabio and Philip H. Gordon[1]
Division of Colon and Rectal Surgery, Sir Mortimer B. Davis – Jewish General Hospital, McGill University, Montreal, Quebec, Canada.

ABSTRACT

Hemorrhoidal disease is the consequence of pathological changes of fibrovascular anal cushions producing symptoms. Symptomatic hemorrhoids may present with bleeding, prolapse, pruritus, soiling, thrombosis and pain. All the potential differential diagnoses of hemorrhoidal disease must be considered in the diagnostic process, as many different colorectal diseases may cause overlapping signs and symptoms.

Treatment includes conservative management (dietary management and lifestyle modifications), which may be effective in the treatment of grade I and some grade II hemorrhoids. Patients still reporting symptoms after conservative management may be candidates for minimally invasive office procedures. These are recommended for most patients with refractory grade I, grade II or grade III hemorrhoids. Surgical hemorrhoidectomy is the treatment of choice for grade IV hemorrhoids, strangulated hemorrhoids and some symptomatic grade III hemorrhoids. Surgical excision is also indicated when minimally invasive office procedures fail to relieve hemorrhoidal

[1]Correspondence: Philip H. Gordon, M.D., FRCS(C), FACS. Sir Mortimer B. Davis – Jewish General Hospital, 3755 Cote Ste. Catherine Road, Montreal, Quebec, Canada H3T 1E2, Phone: +1-514-342-1772, Fax: +1-514-340-7560, E-mail: philip.gordon@mcgill.ca.

symptoms and when patients are not able to tolerate office procedures. Only 5-10% of patients require surgery. Surgical hemorrhoidectomy is considered the most effective treatment for hemorrhoids with fewer recurrences. However, it is associated with more pain and postoperative disability compared to minimally invasive office procedures.

INTRODUCTION

Hemorrhoids have classically been defined as pathologically dilated veins of the lower rectum, but this is not a precise definition. Hemorrhoidal tissue is normally present in the anorectal anatomy. It is composed of cushions of blood vessels, smooth muscle (Treitz's muscle) and connective tissue in the subepithelial space of the anal canal [1]. In addition, the hemorrhoidal blood vessels are not veins, as they do not have muscular wall, but sinusoids with arteriovenous communications. In fact, hemorrhoidal bleeding is arterial and not venous, and is therefore commonly bright red in color [2].

There are three anal fibrovascular cushions which are located in the left lateral, right anterior and right posterior positions of the anus. Smaller secondary cushions may be present between the main cushions [2].

Symptomatic hemorrhoids represent a relevant medical and social problem in the United States, with a prevalence rate of approximately 4%. There are 1.5 million prescriptions per year for medical preparations and a hospitalization rate of 12.9 patients with hemorrhoids per million people. The prevalence of hemorrhoids is equal in men and women, with the highest distribution between age 45 and 65 years [3].

CLASSIFICATION

Hemorrhoids are classified into external and internal (Figure 1). External hemorrhoids are formed by the dilated fibrovascular plexus that is located below the dentate line and covered by squamous epithelium. The internal hemorrhoids are enlarged submucosal fibrovascular tissue located above the dentate line and covered by transitional and columnar epithelium.

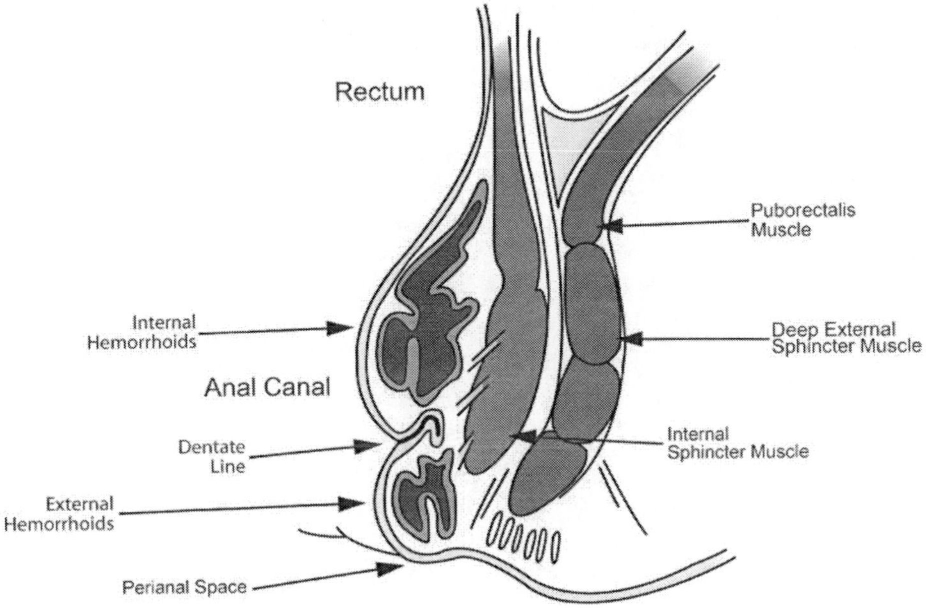

Figure 1. Longitudinal-lateral view of the low rectum and anal canal (schematic representation). External hemorrhoids comprise the symptomatic dilated vascular plexus located below the dentate line and covered by squamous epithelium. Internal hemorrhoids are the symptomatic dilated submucosal vascular tissue located above the dentate line and covered by transitional and columnar epithelium.

Internal hemorrhoids can be divided into four categories based on prolapse and symptoms: grade I internal hemorrhoids bulge into the lumen of the anal canal and may produce painless bleeding; grade II internal hemorrhoids prolapse with straining but reduce spontaneously; grade III internal hemorrhoids protrude spontaneously or with straining and require manual replacement; grade IV internal hemorrhoids are permanently prolapsed and irreducible. Internal and external hemorrhoids may form a combined hemorrhoidal complex (mixed hemorrhoids), as vascular interconnections exist at the dentate line [4].

Etiology and Pathophysiology

Hemorrhoidal tissue is a normal part of the human anorectal anatomy contributing to anal continence and preventing damage to the sphincter mechanism during defecation. Normally, when there is an increase in abdominal pressure (e.g. straining, coughing or sneezing) the anal cushions engorge and maintain closure of the anal canal to prevent leakage of stool. At the time of a bowel movement, the fibrovascular cushions protect the anal canal and allow it to dilate without tearing [2,5].

Hemorrhoidal disease is the consequence of pathological changes of these fibrovascular anal cushions producing symptoms. Although the causes are still unclear, we may identify predisposing or associated factors. Repeated straining during constipation, diarrhea or tenesmus, as well as spending long periods reading on the commode, may induce sliding of the fibrovascular cushions into the anal canal. This may lead to trauma of the internal hemorrhoids with bleeding and progressively to prolapse [6]. If the prolapse persist over time, the continence function may be impaired resulting in mucoid discharge, pruritus and fecal soiling. Other predisposing factors are also prolonged walking, heavy lifting and pregnancy, as a consequence of increased abdominal pressure. Other factors implicated in the causation of hemorrhoidal disease are heredity, absence of valves in the hemorrhoidal plexus and draining veins, and portal hypertension [1].

SYMPTOMS

Symptomatic hemorrhoids may present with bleeding, prolapse, pruritus, soiling, thrombosis and pain.

External hemorrhoids are covered with anoderm innervated with sensory nerve endings. Pain sensation in the anal canal can be felt from the anal verge to 1.5 cm proximal to the dentate line [7]. For this reason, thrombosis of external hemorrhoid is commonly associated with painful perianal lump, which may evolve into a skin tag.

Bleeding is more frequently a consequence of internal hemorrhoids, usually painless bright red bleeding which occurs at the end of defecation. Blood may be present on the tissue paper, on the stool or dripping into the toilet bowl. The bleeding may also be occult, leading in rare cases to anemia [8] or more frequently to guaiac-positive stools. In this circumstance, different causes of bowel bleeding must be excluded before these problems are attributed to hemorrhoids.

Prolapse is commonly due to internal hemorrhoids sliding into the anal canal at the time of defecation. Initially, spontaneous reduction occurs, then manual replacement is necessary, and finally in the advanced cases the prolapse is irreducible. Chronic prolapse predisposes to mucous and fecal leakage that induces pruritus and excoriation of the perianal skin. Hemorrhoids that remain prolapsed may became strangulated and lead to significant edema or gangrene causing pain and occasionally systemic illness. Over time, prolapsed internal hemorrhoids may be associated with external hemorrhoids (combined or mixed hemorrhoids).

DIAGNOSIS

Patients that are referred to the specialist colorectal surgeon for "hemorrhoids" should be carefully evaluated, as many different colorectal diseases may cause overlapping signs and symptoms. At first, careful evaluation of the symptoms should include: characterization of bleeding, pain, mucosal protrusion, mucus discharge, assessment of bowel habits, sensation of incomplete evacuation, or difficulties with perianal hygiene. The initial general assessment must determine whether other disorders such as bleeding disorders, liver disease, portal hypertension, inflammatory bowel diseases or immunosoppression are present. Then, a dietary and medication history should be obtained.

The patient should ideally be examined in a prone position on a special proctological table. Alternatively, the modified left lateral decubitus (Sims) position is also acceptable. The examination should include: anal inspection, digital rectal examination, anoscopy and flexible sigmoidoscopy.

All the potential differential diagnoses of hemorrhoidal disease must be considered in the diagnostic process: anal fissure, fistula, abscess, colorectal polyps/carcinomas, perianal melanoma, perianal endometrioma, inflammatory bowel diseases (in particular perianal Crohn's disease), hypertrophic anal papilla, rectal prolapse, perianal and anal canal condylomata and hidradenitis suppurativa (Table 1).

Anal pain without thrombosed hemorrhoids is more likely a sign of other conditions, such as anal fissure or anorectal abscess.

Rectal bleeding should be carefully evaluated, since it may also be caused by a proximal colorectal neoplasia. Most sources of bright red bleeding are within the reach of a flexible sigmoidoscope, therefore young patients with rectal bleeding and hemorrhoidal disease on examination and no family history of colorectal neoplasia should undergo anoscopy and flexible sigmoidoscopy. In the case of rectal bleeding in an individual older than 50 years [9], or older than 40 years with either a family history [10] of colorectal cancer or a change in bowel habits, a colonoscopy, virtual colonoscopy or barium enema with flexible sigmoidoscopy are required [11].

Table 1. Differential diagnosis of hemorrhoids

Other Diseases	Symptoms
Fissure	Pain, bleeding
Fistula/Abscess	Pain, itching/discharge, bleeding, mass
Colon and rectal polyps/carcinomas	Bleeding, mass
Perianal melanoma	Bleeding, lump/mass
Perianal endometrioma	Mass
Inflammatory bowel diseases (in particular perianal Crohn's disease)	Chronic pain, itching/discharge, mass
Hypertrophic anal papilla	Itching/discharge, lump/mass
Rectal prolapse	Itching/discharge
Perianal and anal canal condylomata acuminata	Itching/discharge
Hidradenitis suppurativa	Itching/discharge, pain

TREATMENT

1) Conservative Management

Dietary management and lifestyle modifications are effective in the treatment of grade I and some grade II hemorrhoids [12].

The primary goal is to have adequate fluid and fiber intake to eliminate straining at defecation and consequently prevent bleeding. A proper diet should include an abundance of fruits and vegetables. Bulk in the diet may be added with raw unprocessed wheat or oat bran (1/3 cup per day). Alternatively, fiber supplement such as psyllium seed (two teaspoons per day), together with adequate water, add moisture to stool and decrease constipation [1]. On rare occasions, psyllium seed may cause an allergic reaction [13]. Stool softeners may also be used. Sitz baths in warm water are useful for anal hygiene and for relieving anal pain [14,15], and should be done two or three times a day. They may also be done at the work place using a portable bowl.

Patients should be educated not to spend long periods of time reading on the toilette bowl, and sometimes by simply changing this habit symptoms may resolve. Patients should also be instructed not to ignore the urge to defecate.

Many topical agents, suppositories and creams are available to alleviate local pain, irritation and pruritus. Most are of marginal if any benefit. Preparations (particularly those containing corticosteroids) should be used for a limited amount of time (e.g. one week), since they may cause mucosal atrophy with ulceration of the perianal skin [11].

Oral venotonics, such as flavonoids, have been used in the treatment of symptomatic hemorrhoids. However, their actual efficacy remains unclear [16].

2) Outpatient and Minor Procedures (Minimally Invasive Procedures)

Patients still reporting symptoms after conservative management may be candidates for minimally invasive procedures that may be performed in the office. These are recommended for most patients with refractory grade I, grade II or grade III hemorrhoids. Patients with grade IV and some with grade III hemorrhoids require definitive surgical treatment, however often at the price of more pain and time away from work.

RUBBER BAND LIGATION

Rubber band ligation is considered the most common office procedure for the treatment of symptomatic grade I, grade II, and selected grade III and grade IV hemorrhoids. The technique is simple, quick and effective [17]. Through an anoscope using a rubber band ligator, a single o double elastic band is fired from the drum onto the redundant rectal mucosa at the top of the internal hemorrhoids (retracted with an atraumatic clamp). The banded tissue becomes necrotic and sloughs off over the next 7-10 days, resulting in a small ulcer. The elastic band must be placed proximal to the dentate line (usually 2 cm). Misplaced rubber band ligation too close to the dentate line can cause severe post treatment pain and may require immediate removal.

Several authors suggest performing ligation at one site at a time, and repeating it at variable intervals of four to six weeks [1]. The rationale of this approach is to reduce postoperative complications such as pain, vaso-vagal symptoms and to facilitate ulcer healing. However, some studies have shown no increase in complication rates with multiple bandings at each visit [18-20].

Symptom relief after rubber band ligation is achieved in 65-85% of patients.

Recurrence of symptoms at 4-5 years of follow-up is approximately 68%, but symptoms usually respond to repeat ligations [21]. It has been estimated that only 5-10% of such patients will require surgical hemorrhoidectomy [11].

Reported complications after rubber band ligation are: pain, bleeding, thrombosis and sepsis. Pain is the most frequent complaint (5-60%) but is usually minor and can easily be relieved with warm sitz bath and analgesics [21,22]. Bleeding may occur immediately after banding or 1-2 weeks after treatment when the eschar from the band sloughs off, and may require surgical intervention with suture ligation. Thrombosis of internal and external hemorrhoids may occasionally arise after rubber band ligation, causing significant pain. Very rarely, cases of perianal sepsis after rubber band ligation have been reported. For this reason this procedure should never be performed in patients with immunodeficiencies [23].

Doppler- Guided Hemorrhoidal Artery Ligation

Doppler-guided hemorrhoidal artery ligation (DGHAL) is performed using a specially designed proctosope (Moricorn) housing a Doppler transducer that can identify hemorrhoidal arteries, and permit their ligation with sutures [24]. DGHAL is a relatively painless method to treat hemorrhoids with low morbidity and a reported success rate as high as 90% for grade III hemorrhoids [24-28]. This procedure is mainly indicated for grade II and grade III hemorrhoids. The failure rate for grade IV hemorrhoids is nearly 70%. The majority of patients undergoing DGHAL require general anesthesia or regional block. Recently, a more complete DGHAL allowing rectoanal repair by mucopexy (DGHAL-RAR) has been developed. These techniques may be regarded as a safe bridge to surgical hemorrhoidectomy for reducible hemorrhoidal prolapse not responding to office procedures, such as rubber band ligation [29]. More studies assessing DGHAL efficacy and long-term results are warranted to prove its efficacy.

Electrocoagulation

Monopolar coagulation may be used with the ball-tip or the spatula-tip. For some authors it is an alternative to rubber band ligation for the treatment of grade II or early grade III hemorrhoids [1,30]. The tops of internal hemorrhoids are coagulated until they are charred, so the mucosa will ulcerate as in the rubber band ligation and fix it to the anorectal ring.

Bipolar (Bicap) coagulation is a form of electrocautery in which heat does not penetrate as deeply as with monopolar coagulation [31]. It is simple to use on an outpatient basis. Bipolar coagulation does not eliminate prolapsing tissue, and up to 20% of patients require excisional hemorrhoidectomy.

Direct current therapy (Ultroid) uses current applied through a probe placed via an anoscope onto the mucosa at the apex of the hemorrhoid. It is a time consuming method, and for this reason has never become popular.

Infrared Photocoagulation

The infrared photocoagulator produces infrared radiation promoting coagulation of vessel and fixation of hemorrhoidal tissue. This procedure is only useful for the treatment of grade I and some grade II hemorrhoids. Compared to rubber band ligation, infrared coagulation has been found to be significantly less painful, but necessitates more sessions to relieve symptoms, has a higher recurrence rate and is more expensive [32,33]. In general, it is not widely used among colorectal surgeons.

SCLEROTHERAPY

Hemorrhoidal sclerotherapy is performed by injecting sclerosant chemical agents into hemorrhoids to create fibrosis and circumvent prolapse. The injection must be made into the submucosa above the internal hemorrhoid at the anorectal ring, and not intravascularly. Sclerotherapy commonly produces pain lasting 48 hours. Misplacement of the injection can lead to mucosal ulceration and necrosis. Sclerotherapy was previously one of the treatments of choice for grade I and grade II hemorrhoids, but currently more effective procedures such as rubber band ligation and electrocoagulation are preferred [1,34,35].

CRYOTHERAPY

Cryotherapy is based on the concept that freezing at low temperature (with nitrous oxide or liquid nitrogen) can destroy the hemorrhoidal cushions. However, due to a high rate of complications, such as irritation, pain due to necrosis, discharge with a foul smell, delayed wound healing and risk of anal stenosis or incontinence, cryotherapy is no longer recommended for the treatment of internal hemorrhoids [1].

3) Surgical Treatment

Surgical hemorrhoidectomy is the treatment of choice for grade IV hemorrhoids, strangulated hemorrhoids (see "special situations" section) and some symptomatic grade III hemorrhoids. Surgical excision is also indicated when minimally invasive procedures fail to relieve hemorrhoidal symptoms and when patients are not able to tolerate office procedures. Only 5-10% of patients require surgery [11]. Surgical hemorrhoidectomy is considered the most effective treatment for hemorrhoids with lower recurrences, but it is associated with more pain and postoperative disability compared to office procedures.

OPEN HEMORRHOIDECTOMY WITH EXCISION AND LIGATION

Open hemorrhoidectomy with excision and ligation is also called Milligan-Morgan hemorrhoidectomy. The procedure is performed with the patient in the lithotomy position. Each hemorrhoid is excised from the underlying sphincter muscle and the pedicle is stick-tied. The skin is left open and heals secondarily in four to eight weeks [36-38]. This procedure is historically mostly performed in the United Kingdom.

Closed Hemorrhoidectomy

Closed hemorrhoidectomy is performed with the patient in the prone jack-knife position. The key to this technique is using the Fansler anal speculum (3 cm in diameter and 7 cm long), which allows excellent exposure of the entire hemorrhoidal tissue. External and internal hemorrhoids are excised from the perianal skin to the anorectal ring. The strip of the excision should not be wider than 1.5 cm. The entire wound is closed with a running rapid absorbable synthetic suture. When a three-quadrant hemorrhoidectomy is planned, it is preferable to first excise the most redundant hemorrhoid and analyse the result. In some circumstances a two-quadrant hemorrhoidectomy may be sufficient [1], allowing the preservation of some anal cushion and the maintainance of good anal continence.

Both open and closed hemorrhoidectomies have been shown to be equally effective. No major differences with respect to postoperative pain, analgesic use, hospital stay and complication were found in clinical trials [39-42]. Closed hemorrhoidectomy seems to promote faster wound healing.

LigaSure™ and Harmonic Scalpel™ Hemorrhoidectomy

LigaSure™ [43,44] and Harmonic Scalpel™ [45-48] have recently been evaluated for use in hemorrhoidectomy. Only LigaSure™ seems to offer some advantages. However, the main limiting factor against the routine use of these instruments is their high cost and the lack of relevant studies analyzing long-term control of hemorrhoidal symptoms.

Stapled Hemorrhoidopexy

Stapled hemorrhoidopexy is a relatively new technique developed to treat prolapsed hemorrhoids. It was popularized by Antonio Longo of the University of Palermo, Italy, in 1998 [49]. In the literature it is also known as: stapled hemorrhoidectomy, stapled anopexy, circumferential mucosectomy, rectal prolapsectomy, circular hemorrhoidectomy, circumferential stapled anoplasty, and stapled rectal mucosectomy. In 2001 an expert panel came up with the official term stapled hemorrhoidopexy [50]. With this procedure prolapsing hemorrhoidal tissue is resuspended back into the anal canal. The hemorrhoids are not removed but repositioned in their original anatomic location. This is done with a 33 mm stapling gun which performs a circumferential resection of mucosa and submucosa above the hemorrhoids and then staples closed the defect [1,11]. The procedure can be executed under local, general or regional anesthesia [1].

The rationale behind stapled hemorrhoidopexy and rubber band ligation does not differ substantially. In both techniques the redundant internal mucosa at the top of the internal hemorrhoid is ligated [11]. Stapled hemorrhoidopexy resects a much larger redundant mucosa and thus would be indicated for severe grade III or grade IV hemorrhoids. Prolapsed internal hemorrhoids that are fixed or immobile are not suitable for the stapled procedure [51].

Stapled hemorrhoidopexy is safe, effective, rapid, and performed with minimal pain in most patients [52-54]. However, it requires proper training and experience in anorectal surgery and with circular stapling devices [1]. Severe complications have been reported in the literature, including: postoperative bleeding, persistent pain, anal sphincter injuries, rectal perforation, retroperitoneal sepsis, anovaginal fistula and pelvic sepsis. Bleeding from the staple line is quite common, and usually requires additional stitches. The other complications are likely to be due to excision of full-thickness rectal wall rather than mucosa and submucosa only [1,11].

The relatively high cost of the equipment may be one major reason why stapled hemorrhoidopexy is not performed on a large scale. Further well designed and adequately powered randomized controlled trials (RCT) are necessary for establishing the cost-effectiveness and long-term efficacy of stapled hemorrhoidopexy. The technique is not universally adopted by many established surgeons.

Other Types of Hemorrhoidectomy

Laser hemorrhoidectomy is performed using a Nd:YAG laser or carbon dioxide laser. This procedure generated some enthusiasm in the past. To date, it does not seem to offer any significant advantages compared to other approaches, and the required equipment is expensive [55-57].

Whitehead hemorrhoidectomy is performed by excision of the submucosal and subdermal hemorrhoidal plexuses circumferentially at the dentate line. The main indication of Whitehead hemorrhoidectomy is for extensive circumferential hemorrhoids. However, severe late complications such as stenosis and ectropion have been reported. Only surgeons very familiar with the technique should perform this procedure to avoid serious consequences [58].

Early Postoperative Problems

Early postoperative problems tend to be more common after surgical hemorrhoidectomy and are summarized as follows: pain, urinary retention, urinary tract infection, postoperative bleeding, fecal impaction, and very rarely perineal and retroperitoneal sepsis [1,23].

Pain is extremely common after hemorrhoidectomy [1]. For this reason it is necessary to prescribe a non-codeine containing oral analgesic. Since the local pain may be partially caused by the spasm of the internal sphincter, topical diltiazem ointment has been suggested to offer some benefit in reducing the pain [59].

Urinary retention (2-36%) and urinary catheterization may be prevented by restricting intravenous fluid to about 500 mL, and limiting postoperative fluid intake [1]. Also warm sitz baths and analgesics may lessen urinary retention. Urinary tract infection (5%) may be a consequence of urinary retention [60].

Postoperative bleeding within 24-48 hours after surgery is usually due to a technical cause. The hemorrhoidal wounds should be closed with continuous sutures [1].

Fecal impaction is a serious complication after hemorrhoidectomy and should be prevented. Patients must be encouraged to eat a high-fiber diet with supplements of psyllium and water. If no bowel movement has occurred after the second postoperative day, a mild laxative plus adequate fluids are required. If the problem persists, manual disimpaction with anesthesia may be necessary.

Infection is extremely uncommon after surgery for hemorrhoids (less than 1%) [60]. However, all the minimally invasive and surgical procedures may potentially be complicated by severe sepsis. Perineal sepsis should be suspected with severe perineal or abdominal pain, persisting urinary retention or difficulties with micturition, fever and leucocytosis. Treatment options for perineal sepsis include antibiotics, prompt drainage, and surgical debridement if necessary. Should Fournier's gangrene supervene, fecal diversion may be required. [23]. Retroperitoneal sepsis manifests with retroperitoneal gas and purulent fluid. In this circumstance, it is reasonable to treat with antibiotics as a first option, given the fact that surgery seems to offer only a limited advantage [23].

Evidence-Based Surgery

1) Comparison between Excisional Hemorrhoidectomy and Rubber Band Ligation

Rubber band ligation is probably the most used minimally invasive office procedure and may be considered an alternative to excisional hemorrhoidectomy for the treatment of grade III hemorrhoids. The technique selection must take into account both the patient's preference and the short- and long-term results of the two procedures that emerge from the literature. The comparison between the therapeutic efficacy of rubber band ligation and excisional hemorrhoidectomy for the treatment of symptomatic hemorrhoids has been the subject of a Cochrane systematic review by Shanmugam et al. (2005), including 3 RCT [61]. The authors found that in the long-term, patients undergoing excisional hemorrhoidectomies have fewer than 20% symptom recurrence and significantly fewer re-treatments compared to rubber band ligation. This difference was more evident for grade II than grade III hemorrhoids. In the short-term, more patients undergoing excisional hemorrhoidectomy experienced postoperative pain. Time off from work was significantly less following rubber band ligation than excisional hemorrhoidectomy.

No significant difference in the incidence of postoperative complications such as urinary retention, postoperative hemorrhage, anal stenosis, acute anal fissure, or fecal incontinence was detected between the two techniques. However, after performing data sub-analyses, the overall delayed complications rate was significantly higher among patients treated with excisional hemorrhoidectomy. No difference in overall early complications rate was found. Data comparing quality of life and economic consequences of either treatment are lacking.

The patient with grade III hemorrhoids willing to undergo surgery should be informed of the long-term efficacy of excisional hemorrhoidectomy but also of the risk of increased postoperative pain compared to rubber band ligation. We still need studies focusing on the health economic evaluation of the two procedures, considering the increased re-treatment rate and repeat time off from work associated with rubber band ligation [61].

2) Comparison between Conventional Surgical Hemorrhoidectomy and Stapled Hemorrhoidopexy

Two recent major systematic reviews summarize well the debate on the efficacy and safety of stapled hemorrhoidopexy compared to the well established conventional surgery for hemorrhoids.

A Cochrane review by Jayaraman et al. (2006) including 12 RCT [62] found that both conventional hemorrhoidectomy and stapled hemorrhoidopexy are safe procedures with very few complications reported. With regard to clinical outcomes, stapled hemorrhoidopexy is associated with a higher long-term risk of hemorrhoid recurrence and higher rates of prolapse symptoms. Consequently, patients undergoing stapled hemorrhoidopexy are more likely to require additional operations compared to those undergoing conventional excisional hemorrhoid surgeries. No significant difference regarding pain in favor of stapled hemorrhoidopexy was found. The authors concluded that: "If hemorrhoid recurrence and prolapse are the most important clinical outcomes, the conventional excisional surgery remains the gold standard in the surgical treatment of internal hemorrhoids" [62].

Burch et al. (2009) included in their systematic review 27 RCT [63]. In addition to clinical outcomes analysis they also included cost assessment, by considering the mean cost of the initial hospital admission, mean operating time and length of stay, the unit cost of a day in hospital, and the surgical costs. They found that stapled hemorrhoidopexy resulted in less pain in the postoperative period, but a higher rate of prolapse and the need for additional operations for prolapse in the long term. There was no difference in the complication rate between the two procedures. Interestingly, the difference in hospital costs was only £9, where additional cost of the staple gun was offset by saving in operating time and hospital stay. The authors concluded that: "The decision to conduct stapled hemorrhoidopexy or conventional hemorrhoidectomy should primarily be based upon the priorities and preferences of the patient (short-term reduction in pain and convalescence, or longer term reduced risk of recurrence) and surgeon" [63].

Large, high quality and adequately powered RCT comparing stapled hemorrhoidopexy and conventional hemorrhoidectomy are certainly needed to establish more rigorous indications.

3) Comparison between Conventional Hemorrhoidectomy and Ligasure™ Hemorrhoidectomy

The bipolar electrothermal sealing device or Ligasure™ (Valleylab, Boulder, CO) uses very high frequency current providing hemostasis by denaturating collagen and elastin from the vessel wall and surrounding connective tissue. Ligasure™ has been introduced for hemorrhoidectomy due to its characteristic of minimal collateral thermal spread and limited tissue charring through use of active feedback control over the power output. This may result in a less painful procedure as compared to conventional surgical hemorrhoidectomy. This hypothesis has been evaluated in a recent Cochrane review by Nienhuijs and de Hingh (2009) including 12 RCT [64]. They found a significant reduction of postoperative pain with Ligasure™ , although this benefit seemed to be reduced two weeks after surgery. The conventional surgical hemorrhoidectomy was associated with more days to return to work. Postoperative complications were similar in both groups.

The efficacy of Ligasure™ will be fully established only when long-term follow-up for evaluation of risk of recurrent hemorrhoidal disease is available. In addition, large scale costs analyses for Ligasure™ are still lacking. If additional costs for the device are taken into account, they could be counterbalanced by general socio-economical aspects, such as earlier return to work [64].

SPECIAL SITUATIONS

Thrombosed External Hemorrhoids

Thrombosis of the external hemorrhoids is characterized by a painful mass in the perianal area (below the dentate line). The pain is described as excruciating or burning. Usually, there is an acute onset of an anal mass and pain that peaks within 48 hours and tends to decrease after the fourth day. Thereafter, the thrombus will shrink and progressively dissolve. A large thrombus may result in a skin tag.

The treatment may be surgical or conservative. If the patient has intense pain, excision of the thrombus produces immediate pain relief, but for maximum benefit the procedure should be performed within the first four days from pain onset [1]. However, if the pain is tolerable, conservative management by using analgesic drugs, warm sitz baths, proper anal hygiene and bulk-forming agents such as bran or psyllium is preferable [1]. Some studies recently showed that nitroglycerine ointment [65] and nifedipine gel [66] may provide temporary analgesia by reducing internal anal sphincter spasm and improving anodermal blood flow.

It is reasonable to suggest a sigmoidoscopy or a colonoscopy, if not recently performed, at the resolution of the symptoms.

Strangulated Hemorrhoids

Strangulated hemorrhoids appear as marked prolapsed and edematous internal and external hemorrhoids. They are the result of prolonged grade 3 or grade 4 hemorrhoidal prolapse on straining. The main symptom is vivid pain which may be associated with urinary retention. Urgent or emergent hemorrhoidectomy is required. If untreated, the edema may progress to ulceration and necrosis with subsequent infection [1].

Hemorrhoids in Pregnancy

The onset or intensification of hemorrhoidal symptoms is a frequent event during pregnancy or vaginal delivery. Hemorrhoidectomy is indicated during pregnancy only in the event of acute prolapse and thrombosis [1]. The operation should be performed under local anesthesia. In the second and third trimester the left lateral position can be used [67].

In most cases, hemorrhoidal symptoms that intensify during vaginal delivery resolve spontaneously. However, if prolapse and thrombosis occur during delivery, a postpartum hemorrhoidectomy may be required for symptom relief.

Hemorrhoids, Anorectal Varices and Portal Hypertension

Anorectal varices are a common event in patients with portal hypertension. This is caused by the portosystemic communications existing in the anorectal canal. Hemorrhoids must be distinguished from anorectal varices, which represent a true consequence of portal hypertension. Unlike esophageal varices, anorectal varices rarely bleed [68].

Anorectal varices occur in the anorectal region, and the site of bleeding is usually above the squamous portion of the anal canal. This bleeding may be treated by ligation of 3-4 columns using absorbable running suture from as high as possible in the rectum to just outside the anus depending on the extent of the varices [69]. There are several other treatment options: stapled hemorrhoidopexy [70], portal decompression via a transhepatic portosystemic shunt (TIPS) [71], ligation of the inferior mesenteric vein [72], or portosystemic shunts.

The incidence of true hemorrhoids in patients with portal hypertension is no greater than in the normal population [73]. However, massive bleeding from prolapsed hemorrhoids in patients with portal hypertension may be life threatening. This most frequently happens during treatment of encephalopathy, since it frequently results in severe diarrhea. In this case coagulopathy must be corrected and diarrhea controlled [1]. Bleeding hemorrhoids should be treated by ligation using absorbable sutures [74]. Hemorrhoidectomy should be reserved as the last option for treating the bleeding.

Hemorrhoids in Inflammatory Bowel Disease

Hemorrhoids may be symptomatic in patients with inflammatory bowel disease as a consequence of diarrhea. The treatment of symptomatic hemorrhoids is usually safe in patients with ulcerative colitis. However, in patients with Crohn's disease, hemorrhoidectomy has been associated with complications that can be as severe as requiring proctectomy [75]. Therefore, hemorrhoidectomy in Crohn's disease is relatively contraindicated, but if necessary it should be performed during a quiescent state.

Hemorrhoids in Leukemia and in the Immunocompromised

Hemorrhoidal problems are a rare event in patients with leukemia, lymphoma or other immunocompromising conditions. The main problem is the high risk of postoperative morbidity when surgical treatment is required [76]. In particular, poor wound healing and anal infection with fever, local pain and tenderness are common complications. Therefore, surgery should be the last possible option for treating hemorrhoidal symptoms in this population.

Conclusion

Surgical hemorrhoidectomy is the most effective treatment for hemorrhoids with fewer recurrences, but it is associated with more pain and postoperative disability compared to office procedures. Selection of the best treatment for relieve hemorrhoidal symptoms should be based upon the priorities and preferences of the patient (short-term reduction in pain and convalescence, or longer-term reduced risk of recurrence) and surgeon. We still need large studies focusing on the health economic evaluation of office vs. surgical procedures.

References

[1] Nivatvongs, S. Hemorrhoids. In: Gordon, PH and Nivatvongs, S editors. Principles and Practice of Surgery for the Colon, Rectum, and Anus. 3rd ed. New York: Informa Healthcare USA, 2007, 143-66.

[2] Thompson, WH. The nature of hemorrhoids. *Br. J. Surg.*, 1975; 62, 542-52.

[3] Johanson, JF; Sonnenberg, A. Temporal changes in the occurrence of hemorrhoids in the United States and England. *Dis. Colon Rectum*, 1991; 34, 585-91.

[4] Cataldo, P; Ellis, CN; Gregorcyk, S; Hyman, N; Buie, WD; Church, J; Cohen, J; Fleshner, P; Kilkenny, J 3rd; Ko, C; Levien, D; Nelson, R; Newstead, G; Orsay, C; Perry, WB; Rakinic, J; Shellito, P; Strong, S; Ternent, C; Tjandra, J; Whiteford, M; The Standards Practice Task Force, The American Society of Colon and Rectal Surgeons, USA. Practice parameters for the management of hemorrhoids (revised). *Dis. Colon Rectum*, 2005; 48, 189-94.

[5] Lestar, B; Penninckx, F; Kerremans, R. The composition of anal basal pressure. An in vivo and in vitro study in man. *Int. J. Colorectal Dis.*, 1989; 4, 118-22.

[6] Loder, PB; Kamm, MA; Nicholls, RJ; Phillips, RK. Haemorrhoids: pathology, pathophysiolgy and aetiology. *Br. J. Surg.*, 1994; 81, 946-54.

[7] Schouten, WR; Gordon, PH. Physiology. In: Gordon, PH and Nivatvongs, S editors. Principles and Practice of Surgery for the Colon, Rectum, and Anus. 3rd ed. New York: Informa Healthcare USA, 2007, 29-64.

[8] Kluiber, RM; Wolff, BG. Evaluation of anemia caused by hemorrhoidal bleeding. *Dis. Colon Rectum*, 1994; 37, 1006-7.

[9] Imperiale, TF; Wagner, DR; Lin, CY; Larkin, GN; Rogge, JD; Ransohoff, DF. Results of screening colonoscopy among persons 40 to 49 years of age. *N. Engl. J. Med.*, 2002; 346, 1781-5.

[10] Winawer, S; Fletcher, R; Rex, D; Bond, J; Burt, R; Ferrucci, J; Ganiats, T; Levin, T; Woolf, S; Johnson, D; Kirk, L; Litin, S; Simmang, C; Gastrointestinal Consortium Panel. Colorectal cancer screening and surveillance: clinical guidelines and rationale-Update based on new evidence. *Gastroenterology,* 2003; 124, 544-60.

[11] Morin, N. American Society of Colon and Rectal Surgeons (ASCRS). 2008 Core Subjects: Hemorrhoids and Fissure-in-Ano. Available from: URL: http://www.fascrs.org/physicians/education/core_subjects/2008/hemorrhoids_fissure_in_ano/

[12] Alonso-Coello, P; Guyatt, G; Heels-Ansdell, D; Johanson, JF; Lopez-Yarto, M; Mills, E; Zhou, Q. Laxatives for the treatment of hemorrhoids. Cochrane Database Syst Rev, 2005 Oct 19;(4):CD004649.

[13] Lantner, RR; Espiritu, BR; Zumerchik, P; Tobin, MC. Anaphylaxis following ingestion of a psyllium-containing cereal. *JAMA,* 1990; 264, 2534-6.

[14] Dodi, G; Bogoni, F; Infantino, A; Pianon, P; Mortellaro, LM; Lise, M. Hot or cold in anal pain? A study of the changes of internal anal sphincter pressure profiles. *Dis. Colon Rectum,* 1986; 29, 248-51.

[15] Shafik, A. Role of warm water bath in anorectal conditions. The "thermosphincteric reflex". *J. Clin. Gastroenterol.,* 1992; 16, 304-8.

[16] Alonso-Coello, P; Zhou, Q; Martinez-Zapata, MJ; Mills, E; Heels-Ansdell, D; Johanson, JF; Guyatt, G. Meta-analysis of flavanoids for the treatment of hemorrhoids. *Br. J. Surg.,* 2006; 93, 909-20.

[17] Iyer, VS; Shrier, I; Gordon, PH. Long-term outcome of rubber band ligation for symptomatic primary and recurrent internal hemorrhoids. *Dis. Colon Rectum,* 2004; 47, 1364-70.

[18] Armstrong, DN. Multiple hemorrhoidal ligation: a prospective, randomized trial evaluating a new technique. *Dis. Colon Rectum*, 2003; 46, 179-86.

[19] Komborozos, VA; Skrekas, GJ; Pissiotis, CA. Rubber band ligation of symptomatic internal hemorrhoids: results of 500 cases. *Dig. Surg.,* 2000; 17, 71-6.

[20] Law, WL; Chu, KW. Triple rubber band ligation for hemorrhoids: prospective, randomized trial of use of local anesthetic injection. *Dis. Colon Rectum,* 1999; 42, 363-6.

[21] Madoff, RD; Fleshman, JW. American Gastroenetrological Association technical review on the diagnosis and treatment of hemorrhoids. *Gastroenterology*, 2004; 126, 1463-73.

[22] Hardwick, RH; Durdey, P. Should rubber band ligation of haemorrhoids be performed at the initial outpatient visit? *Ann. R. Coll .Surg. Engl.,* 1994; 76, 185-7.

[23] McCloud, JM; Jameson, JS; Scott, AN. Life-threatening sepsis following treatment for haemorrhoids: a systematic review. *Colorectal Dis*., 2006; 8, 748-55.

[24] Morinaga, K; Hasuda, K; Ikeda, T. A novel therapy for internal hemorrhoids: ligation of the hemorrhoidal artery with a newly devised instrument (Moricorn) in conjunction with a Doppler flowmeter. *Am. J. Gastroenterol*., 1995; 90, 610-3.

[25] Sohn, N; Aronoff, JS; Cohen, FS; Weinstein, MA. Transanal hemorrhoidal dearterialization is an alternative to operative hemorrhoidectomy. *Am. J. Surg.,* 2001; 182, 515-9.

[26] Ramírez, JM; Aguilella, V; Elía, M; Gracia, JA; Martínez, M. Doppler-guided hemorrhoidal artery ligation in the management of symptomatic hemorrhoids. *Rev. Esp. Enferm. Dig.,* 2005; 97, 97-103.

[27] Felice, G; Privitera, A; Ellul, E; Klaumann, M. Doppler-guided hemorrhoidal artery ligation: An alternative to hemorrhoidectomy. *Dis. Colon Rectum,* 2005; 48, 2090-3

[28] Greenberg, R; Karin, E; Avital, S; Skornick, Y; Werbin, N. First 100 cases with Doppler-guided hemorrhoidal artery ligation. *Dis. Colon Rectum,* 2006; 49, 485-9.

[29] Conaghan, P; Farouk, R. Doppler-guided hemorrhoid artery ligation reduces the need for conventional hemorrhoid surgery in patients who fail rubber band ligation treatment. *Dis. Colon Rectum,* 2009; 52, 127-30.

[30] Randall, GM; Jensen, DM; Machicado, GA; Hirabayashi, K; Jensen, ME; You, S; Pelayo, E. Prospective randomized comparative study of bipolar versus direct current electrocoagulation for treatment of bleeding internal hemorrhoids. *Gastrointest. Endosc*., 1994; 40, 403-10.

[31] Dennison, A; Whiston, RJ; Rooney, S; Chadderton, RD; Wherry, DC; Morris, DL. A randomized comparison of infrared photocoagulation with bipolar diathermy for the outpatient treatment of hemorrhoids. *Dis. Colon Rectum,* 1990; 33, 32-4.

[32] Johanson, JF; Rimm, A. Optimal nonsurgical treatment of hemorrhoids: a comparative analysis of infrared coagulation, rubber band ligation, and injection sclerotherapy. *Am. J. Gastroenterol.,* 1992; 87, 1600-6.

[33] McRae, HM; McLeod, RS. Comparison of hemorrhoidal treatments: a meta-analysis. *Dis. Colon Rectum*, 1995; 38, 687-94.

[34] Alexander-Williams, J; Crapp, AR. Conservative management of haemorrhoids. Part I: injection, freezing and ligation. *Clin. Gastroenterol.*, 1975; 4, 595-618.

[35] Senapati, A; Nicholls, RJ. A randomised trial to compare the results of injection sclerotherapy with a bulk laxative alone in the treatment of bleeding haemorrhoids. *Int. J. Colorectal Dis*., 1988; 3, 124-6.

[36] Milligan, ETC; Morgan, CN; Jones, LE; Officer, R. Surgical anatomy of the anal canal and the operative treatment of hemorrhoids. *Lancet*, 1937; 2, 1119-24.

[37] Andrews, BT; Layer, GT; Jackson, BT; Nicholls, RJ. Randomized trial comparing diathermy hemorrhoidectomy with the scissor dissection Milligan-Morgan operation. *Dis Colon Rectum*, 1993; 36, 580-3.

[38] Seow-Choen, F; Ho, YH; Ang, HG; Goh, HS. Prospective, randomized trial comparing pain and clinical function after conventional scissors excision/ligation vs. diathermy excision without ligation for symptomatic prolapsed hemorrhoids. *Dis. Colon Rectum*, 1992; 35, 1165-9.

[39] Ho, YH; Seow-Choen, F; Tan, M; Leong, AF. Randomized controlled trial of open and closed haemorrhoidectomy. *Br. J. Surg.,* 1997; 84, 1729-30.

[40] Carapeti, EA; Kamm, MA; McDonald, PJ; Chadwick, SJ; Phillips, RK. Randomized trial of open versus closed day-case haemorrhoidectomy. *Br. J. Surg.,* 1999; 86, 612-3.

[41] Arbman, G; Krook, H; Haapaniemi, S. Closed vs. open hemorrhoidectomy-is there any difference? *Dis. Colon Rectum*, 2000; 43, 31-4.

[42] Gecosmanoglu, R Sad O; Koc, D; Inceoglu, R. Hemorrhoidectomy: open or closed technique? A prospective, randomized clinical trial. *Dis. Colon Rectum,* 2002; 45, 70-5.

[43] Palazzo, FF; Francis, DL; Clifton, MA. Randomized clinical trial of Ligasure versus open haemorrhoidectomy. *Br. J. Surg*., 2002; 89, 154–7.

[44] Jayne, DG; Botterill, I; Ambrose, NS; Brennan, TG; Guillou, PJ; O'Riordain, DS. Randomized clinical trial of Ligasure versus conventional diathermy for day-case hemorrhoidectomy. *Br. J. Surg*., 2002; 89, 428-32.

[45] Khan, S; Pawlak, SE; Eggenberger, JC; Lee, CS; Szilagy, EJ; Wu, JS; Margolin, M D DA. Surgical treatment of hemorrhoids: prospective, randomized trial comparing closed excisional hemorrhoidectomy and the

Harmonic Scalpel technique of excisional hemorrhoidectomy. *Dis. Colon Rectum*, 2001; 44, 845-9.

[46] Tan, JJ; Seow-Choen, F. Prospective, randomized trial comparing diathermy and Harmonic scalpel hemorrhoidectomy: a prospective evaluation. *Dis. Colon Rectum*, 2001; 44, 677-79.

[47] Armstrong, DN; Ambroze, WL; Schertzer, ME; Orangio, GR. Harmonic scalpel vs. electrocautery hemorrhoidectomy: a prospective evaluation. *Dis. Colon Rectum*, 2001; 44, 558-64.

[48] Chung, CC; Ha, JP; Tai, YP; Tsang, WW; Li, MK. Double- blind, randomized trial comparing Harmonic Scalpel hemorrhoidectomy, bipolar scissors hemorrhoidectomy, and scissors excision: ligation technique. *Dis. Colon Rectum*, 2002; 45, 789-94.

[49] Longo, A. Treatment of hemorrhoidal disease by reduction of mucosa and hemorrhoidal prolapse with a circular suturing device: a new procedure. Proceeding of the 6th world congress of endoscopic surgery, Rome, 1998, 777-84.

[50] Corman, ML; Gravié, JF; Hager, T; Loudon, MA; Mascagni, D; Nyström, PO; Seow-Choen, F; Abcarian, H; Marcello, P; Weiss, E; Longo, A. Stapled haemorrhoidopexy: a consensus position paper by an international working party - indications, contra-indications and technique. *Colorectal Dis.*, 2003; 5, 304-10.

[51] Ortiz, H; Marzo, J; Armendáriz, P; De Miguel, M. Stapled hemorrhoidopexy vs. diathermy excision for fourth-degree hemorrhoids: a randomized, clinical trial and review of the literature. *Dis. Colon Rectum*, 2005; 48, 809 15.

[52] Singer, MA; Cintron, JR; Fleshman, JW; Chaudhry, V; Birnbaum, EH; Read, TE; Spitz, JS; Abcarian, H. Early experience with stapled hemorrhoidectomy in the United States. *Dis. Colon Rectum*, 2002; 45, 360-7.

[53] Arnaud, JP; Pessaux, P; Huten, N; De Manzini, N; Tuech, JJ; Laurent, B; Simone, M. Treatment of hemorrhoids with circular stapler, a new alternative to conventional methods: a prospective study of 140 patients. *J. Am. Coll. Surg.*, 2001; 193, 161-5.

[54] Habr-Gama, A; e Sous, AH Jr; Roveló, JM; Souza, JV; Benício, F; Regadas, FS; Wainstein, C; da Cunha, TM; Marques, CF; Bonardi, R; Ramos, JR; Pandini, LC; Kiss, D. Stapled hemorrhoidectomy: initial experience of a Latin American group. *J. Gastrointest. Surg.*, 2003; 7, 809-13.

[55] Wang, JY; Chang-Chien, CR; Chen, JS; Lai, CR; Tang, RP. The role of lasers in hemorrhoidectomy. *Dis. Colon Rectum*, 1991; 34, 78–82.

[56] Iwagaki, H; Higuchi, Y; Fuchimoto, S; Orita, K. The laser treatment of hemorrhoids: results of a study on 1816 patients. *Jpn. J. Surg.*, 1989; 19, 658–61.

[57] Senagore, A; Mazier, WP; Luchtefeld, MA; MacKeigan, JM; Wengert, T. Treatment of advanced hemorrhoidal disease: a prospective, randomized comparison of cold scalpel vs. contact Nd:YAG laser. *Dis. Colon Rectum*, 1993; 36, 1042–9.

[58] Wolff, BG; Culp, CE. The Whitehead hemorrhoidectomy. An unjustly maligned procedure. *Dis. Colon Rectum*, 1988; 31, 587-90.

[59] Silverman, R; Bendick, PJ; Wasvary, HJ. A randomized, prospective, double-blind, placebo-controlled trial of the effect of a calcium channel blocker ointment on pain after hemorrhoidectomy. *Dis. Colon Rectum*, 2005; 48, 1913-6

[60] Bleday, R; Pena, JP; Rothenberger, DA; Goldberg, SM; Buls, JG. Symptomatic hemorrhoids: current incidence and complications of operative therapy. *Dis. Colon Rectum*, 1992; 35, 477-81.

[61] Shanmugam, V; Thaha, MA; Rabindranath, KS; Campbell, KL; Steele, RJ; Loudon, MA. Rubber band ligation versus excisional haemorrhoidectomy for haemorrhoids. Cochrane Database Syst Rev, 2005 Jul 20;(3):CD005034.

[62] Jayaraman, S; Colquhoun, PH; Malthaner, RA. Stapled versus conventional surgery for hemorrhoids. *Cochrane Database Syst. Rev.*, 2006 Oct 18;(4):CD005393.

[63] Burch, J; Epstein, D; Sari, AB; Weatherly, H; Jayne, D; Fox, D; Woolacott, N. Stapled haemorrhoidopexy for the treatment of haemorrhoids: a systematic review. *Colorectal Dis.*, 2009; 11, 233-43.

[64] Nienhuijs, S; de Hingh, I. Conventional versus LigaSure hemorrhoidectomy for patients with symptomatic Hemorrhoids. *Cochrane Database Syst. Rev.*, 2009 Jan 21;(1):CD006761.

[65] Gorfine, SR. Treatment of benign anal disease with topical nitroglycerin. *Dis. Colon Rectum*, 1995; 38, 453-6.

[66] Perrotti, P; Antropoli, C; Noschese, G; Bartone, G; De Stefano, G; Pacifico, F; Maffettone, A; Antropoli, M. Topical nifedipine for conservative treatment of acute hemorrhoidal thrombosed. *Colorectal Dis.*, 2000; 2, 18-21.

[67] Nivatvongs, S. Alternative positioning of patients for hemorrhoidectomy. *Dis Colon Rectum*, 1980; 23, 308-9.

[68] Johansen, K; Bardin, J; Orloff, MJ. Massive bleeding from hemorrhoidal varices in portal hypertension. *JAMA,* 1980; 244, 2084-5.
[69] Hosking, SW; Johnson, AG. Bleeding anorectal varices--a misunderstood condition. *Surgery*, 1988; 104, 70-3.
[70] Biswas, S; George, ML; Leather, AJ. Stapled anopexy in the treatment of anal varices: report of a case. *Dis. Colon Rectum*, 2003; 46, 1284-5.
[71] Katz, JA; Rubin, RA; Cope, C; Holland, G; Brass, CA. Recurrent bleeding from anorectal varices: successful treatment with a transjugular intrahepatic portosystemic shunt. *Am. J. Gastroenterol.*, 1993; 88, 1104-7.
[72] Yeh, T Jr; McGuire, HH Jr. Intractable bleeding from anorectal varices relieved by inferior mesenteric vein ligation. *Gastroenterology*, 1994; 107, 1165-7.
[73] Bernstein, WC. What are hemorrhoids and what is their relationship to the portal venous system? *Dis. Colon Rectum*, 1983; 26, 829-34.
[74] Nivatvongs, S. Suture of massive hemorrhoidal bleeding in portal hypertension. *Dis. Colon Rectum*, 1985; 28, 878-9.
[75] Jeffery, PJ; Parks, AG; Ritchie, JK. Treatment of haemorrhoids in patients with inflammatory bowel disease. *Lancet,* 1977; 1, 1084-5.
[76] Grewal, H; Guillem, JG; Quan, SH; Enker, WE; Cohen, AM. Anorectal disease in neutropenic leukemic patients. Operative vs. nonoperative management. *Dis. Colon Rectum,* 1994; 37, 1095-9.

In: Hemorrhoids: Symptoms, Diagnosis… ISBN: 978-1-60876-478-5
Authors: P. Salinitri et al., pp. 25-54

Chapter 2

TREATMENT OF HEMORRHOIDS

Marcello Picchio[1]*, Giuseppe Marino,* Ettore Greco* and Erasmo Spaziani†

* Department of Surgery, Hospital "P. Colombo", Via Orti Ginnetti 7, 00049 Velletri, Rome, Italy

† Department of Surgery, University of Rome "La Sapienza"–Polo Pontino, Hospital "A. Fiorini," Via Firenze, 04019 Terracina, Latina, Italy

ABSTRACT

Hemorrhoids are one of the most frequent pathologies, with an estimated prevalence of 4.4%. Treatment strategies are various and can be divided into conservative therapies (either paharmacological or instrumental) and surgery.

Medical therapy includes vasoactive agents (flavonoids) and various topical agents aiming to reduce symptoms.

Instrumental therapies (elastic band ligation, sclerotherapy, cryotherapy, cauterization, etc.) can be effective in about 70–90% of patients in the short term with a significant rate of recurrence in the long term.

Surgical therapy guaranties satisfactory results, which are significantly better that those obtained with conservative therapies, especially for grade III and IV hemorrhoids. Traditional surgery for hemorrhoids aims to remove the hemorroids, with closure (Fergusson's technique) or without closure (Milligan-Morgan procedure) of the ensuing defect. This traditional approach is effective, but causes significant postoperative pain because of wide

[1] Correspondence to: Marcello Picchio, MD, Viale Giulio Cesare 58, 04100 – Latina (Italy). Tel.: +39773695488; E.mail: marcellopicchio@libero.it

external wounds in the innervated perianal skin. Stapled hemorrhopidopexy, proposed by Longo, has gained vast acceptance because of less postoperative pain and faster return to normal activities. This technique aims to reduce the hemorrhoidal prolapse by repositioning the hemorrhoidal masses into the anal canal and by reducing the venous engorgement with transaction of feeding arteries and redundant mucosa. The procedure results in a stapled mucosa anastomosis in the rectum, at least 3 cm above the dentate line where sensitive receptors are few, without any dissection or trauma in the area of anal mucosa and anoderm.

The superiority of stapled hemorrhoidopexy in terms of less postoperative pain and quicker recovery was confirmed by a recent systematic review of 25 randomized trials comparing stapled hemorrhoidopexy and conventional hemorrhoidectomy. However, the long-term control of hemorrhoid symptoms as well as the recurrence of prolapsing hemorrhoids should be addressed in order to draw a final conclusion about the efficacy and effectiveness of stapled hemorrhoidopexy. In the recent literature, a significant incidence of recurrence after stapled hemorrhoidopexy was reported. In particular, when compared with conventional hemorrhoidectomy, stapled hemorrhoidopexy resulted in a higher incidence of recurrence and a worse clinical outcome. The higher recurrence rate may be sometimes the result of inappropriate patient selection. Therefore, with the presence of large-volume prolapsing internal hemorrhoids, we could imagine that stapled hemorrhoidopexy using two staplers would not be appropriate. Further prospective studies with more attention to appropriate patient selection are necessary to assess the efficacy of the various surgical procedures for hemorrhoids.

Introduction

Anal cushions are normal structural components of the anal canal, serving as a conformable plug to ensure its complete closure. Hemorrhoids should be considered pathologic when symptomatic prolapse occurs. Hospital-based proctoscopy studies reported the presence of hemorrhoids in up to 86% of patients, even though many of them were asymptomatic [1]. The need for treatment is influenced by the severity of symptoms. Management should aim to control symptoms and can be broadly classified as conservative, alternative and surgical.

CONSERVATIVE THERAPY

Minimizing constipation and the prolonged straining that may be associated are among the main purposes of lifestyle modifications recommended in primary care to manage hemorrhoid disease. The effectiveness of increasing fluid intake as a treatment for constipation remains unknown. Dietary fiber intake may alleviate occasional and moderate constipation [2,3]. A recent meta-analysis confirmed that fiber supplements moderately improve overall symptoms and bleeding and should be recommended in grade I–II hemorrhoids [4]. Because diarrhea exacerbates hemorrhoidal symptoms, controlling it with fiber, antimotility agents and specific treatment of any underlying cause will likely be of benefit. The traditional recommendation to avoid alcohol, spices and pepper is justified because they were recognized as risk factors for hemorrhoidal crisis [5]. Other lifestyle modifications such as improving anal hygiene and taking sitz baths are used in primary care and may help in the treatment and prevention of hemorrhoids, although the evidence for this is lacking.

Medical treatment includes both oral and local drugs. Venotonics represent a group of drugs that may improve venous tone and lymphatic drainage and reduce capillary hyperpermeability by protecting the microcirculation from inflammatory processes. Flavonoids, including diosmin, hidrosmin, hesperidin and rutosides, are the most popular. Micronised purified flavonoid fraction is an oral phlebotropic drug made up of 90% micronised diosmin and 10% flavonoids expressed as hesperidin, particularly favored and marketed in Europe and the Far East. Although flavonoids seem to have a beneficial effect in the treatment of symptomatic hemorrhoids, larger and better designed trials are needed to strengthen the quality of evidence [6]. Calcium dobesilate (calcium 2,5-dihydroxybenzenesulfonate) is a drug with the ability to decrease capillary permeability, platelet aggregation and blood viscosity and to increase lymphatic transport. Together with a high-fiber diet it achieved both improvement of symptoms and reduction of anitis in patients suffering from acute attacks of grade I–II hemorrhoids [7]. There is a variety of topical drugs aiming to alleviate symptoms with different mechanisms. Over-the-counter topical preparations that contain a combination of local anesthetics, corticosteroids, astringents and antiseptics are largely used, although there is no evidence supporting their efficacy. In particular, long-term use of steroid creams should be discouraged because it can permanently damage or cause ulceration of the perianal skin [8]. Topical glyceryl trinitrate is a nitric oxide donor and produces vasodilatation of blood vessels with relaxation of the internal anal sphincter muscle (chemical sphincterotomy). Spasm of the internal anal sphincter may be a factor contributing to symptoms either in patients with hemorrhoids or after surgery. In particular, patients with grade I–II hemorrhoids and high maximum resting anal canal pressure benefit from topical glyceryl trinitrate [9]. After hemorrhoidectomy, both pain decrease and accelerated healing are obtained with the local application of glyceryl trinitrate [10].

Conservative therapies may relieve symptoms in early stages but cannot definitively cure hemorrhoids.

Alternative Therapy

Alternative treatment includes a number of ambulatory interventions that usually do not need anesthetics.

Sclerotherapy

Sclerotherapy consists of injection of sclerosing substances, normally 5% oily phenol, in the submucosa of the proximal part of the hemorrhoidal bulk 1 cm above the dentate line with the aid of a syringe and a proctoscope (Figure 1). It is cheap and easy to perform, but it has a high failure rate. Complications with sclerosants are rare but include local infections, prostatitis, portal pyemia, and erectile dysfunction [11]. Conservative treatment with fiber supplementation may be as effective as injection sclerotherapy [12].

A novel sclerosing agent containing the active ingredient aluminum potassium sulfate was proposed for the treatment of grade III and IV hemorrhoids with early satisfactory results [13].

Cryotherapy

This procedure consists in freezing the external and internal hemorrhoids with liquid nitrogen to –196°C or liquid nitrous oxide to –89°C. The main disadvantage of this technique is the prolonged healing time, with resultant pain and drainage. At present, cryotherapy is substantially disappeared.

Infrared coagulation, bipolar diathermy, direct-current electrotherapy, laser therapy

These procedures all rely on the coagulation, occlusion, and obliteration or sclerosis of the hemorrhoidal vascular pedicle above the level of the anal transition zone.

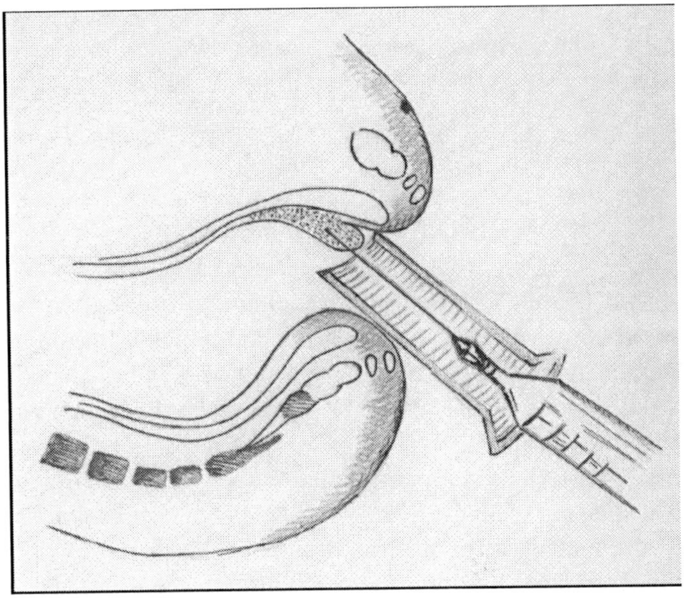

Figure 1. The patient is laid down in the left lateral position. A proctoscope with a wide-bore is inserted into the anal canal to illuminate the hemorrhoid to be injected. Injection should be done at the base of the hemorrhoid, above the dentate line, where no or little pain should be felt. Once the correct injection site is located, the needle is inserted about 1 to 2 cm deep in the submucosal space, parallel to the anal canal. About 3 to 5 ml of sclerosant is injected slowly, allowing time for dispersion in the tissue. Injection should be stopped, if it causes pain. In most patients, a maximum of three separate injections to the base of the hemorrhoids are given.

Infrared photocoagulation consists of coagulating hemorrhoids by means of infrared radiation from a tungsten-halogen lamp via a polymer probe tip. According to two randomized studies, hemorrhoidal bleeding was successfully controlled in 67–96% of patients with first- or second-degree hemorrhoids [14,15]. Complications, including pain and bleeding, are uncommon.

Bipolar diathermy aims to produce tissue destruction by the heat generated by a bipolar probe. It has been used to treat first-, second-, and third-degree internal hemorrhoids with success rates range from 88% to 100% and failure to eliminate prolapse in up to 20% of patients [16].

Direct-current electrotherapy requires the prolonged (up to 14 minutes) application of 110V direct current (up to 15 mA) to the base of the hemorrhoidal complex. A prospective, crossover trial between direct current electrotherapy and medical therapy found no difference [17].

Both Nd:YAG and CO_2 laser have been used to coagulate grade I–II hemorrhoids by using a contact probe. However, its use was not recommended because it may destroy muscles in addition to hemorrhoids with rather disastrous results [18].

Rubber-Band Ligation

Rubber-band ligation is the most commonly used alternative therapy, originally proposed by Blaisdell and later modified by Barron [19,20]. The procedure consists in applying an elastic band at the base of the hemorrhoids, well proximal to the dentate line (Figure 2). At present the commonest practiced technique is the suction method, which makes the procedure a one-person effort. The procedure is performed through a proctoscope, which is inserted and placed about 2 cm above the dentate line. The hemorrhoidal cushion is allowed to prolapse into the lumen of the proctoscope. After introduction of the McGown ligator, suction is applied until the tissue is taut into the drum and the trigger is released expelling a rubber O-ring around the base of the hemorrhoid. The rubber band must be applied at least 1–2 cm above the dentate line. If it is placed too far distally, near the anal transition zone, severe pain usually occurs due to the presence of somatic sensory afferents. The procedure aims to strangulate hemorrhoid, which becomes necrotic and sloughs off, while the underlying tissue undergoes fixation by fibrotic wound healing. The procedure may also be performed using a flexible endoscope with the same technique applied for the treatment of esophageal and gastric varices [21]. The success rates of the method vary, depending on the degree of hemorrhoids treated, length of follow-up, and criteria for success. Wrobleski et al. [22] reported that 80% of their patients improved and 69% were symptom-free at a mean follow-up of 5 years. Steinberg et al. [23] reported 89% patient satisfaction at a similar follow-up interval, but only 44% of their patients were symptom free. Many authors reported that recurrence rate may be as high as 68% at 4 or 5 years of follow-up and symptoms usually respond to repeated ligation, but only 10% of such patients requires excisional hemorrhoidectomy [24,25].

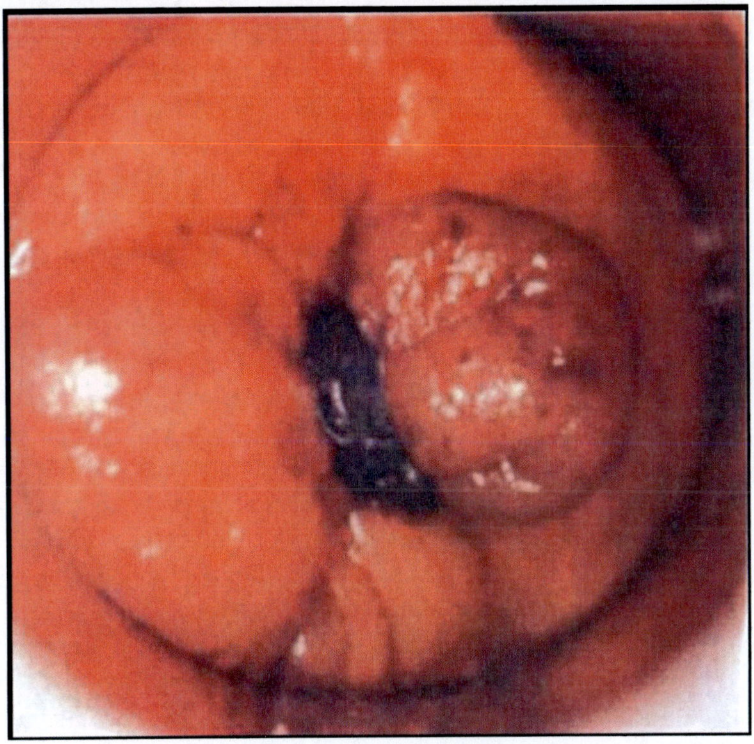

Figure 2. The elastic band is positioned at the base of the hemorrhoid, well proximal to the dentate line.

A review of 39 studies incorporating 8,060 patients undergoing rubber-band ligation showed post-banding complications in the form of severe pain in 5.8%, hemorrhage in 1.7%, infection in 0.05% anal fissure and fistula in 0.4% [26].

CONCLUSION

Two meta-analyses found that rubber-band ligation was more effective than sclerotherapy, less likely to require additional therapy than either sclerotherapy or infrared photocoagulation, and more likely to cause pain [27,28]. When compared with surgery, rubber-band ligation should be adopted as the procedure of choice for grade II hemorrhoids, as it has results similar to those of operation but without the side effects [29].

Combined sclerotherapy and rubber-band ligation was proposed for early hemorrhoids and incomplete mucosal prolapse. The procedure can be performed in an office setting. Each hemorrhoid must be first injected with 5% phenol in almond oil, with subsequent rubber-band ligation. This technique guarantees good results with low rates of recurrence and complications [30].

Each method of alternative therapy was compared with one or more of the others in randomized controlled trials, but adequate studies considering all the techniques are lacking. At present, the exact role of each technique in the treatment of hemorrhoids is still controversial.

SURGICAL THERAPY

Surgery is the most effective treatment for hemorrhoids and is particularly recommended in prolapsing piles during defecation that may be reduced manually (grade III) and irreducible hemorrhoids (grade IV) with respect to nonoperative techniques [28]. Other indications for surgery are failure of nonoperative management, patient preference and concomitant conditions (such as fissure or fistula) that require surgery. Contraindications are generally relative. Surgical option should be carefully proposed if the anesthesiologic risk is high, serious hemostatic and/or coagulative disorders are present, and the presence of anal sphincter and/or continence impairment may lead to postoperative occurrence and/or worsening of incontinence. **Caution is also required if Crohn's disease** is present [31].

PROCEDURES

Numerous methods have been proposed for the surgical therapy of hemorrhoids. Anal dilatation and lateral internal sphincterotomy aimed at relieving the elevated anal sphincter pressure [32,33]. Anal sphincter hypertone was presumed as one of the etiologic factors contributing to the disease [34]. These procedures were abandoned because results were not satisfactory and incontinence was a serious and frequent complication [33,35-37].

Hemorrhoidectomy, performed with various techniques, focuses on resection of both internal and external hemorrhoids and ligature of the main supplying vessels. The rationale of these procedures is based on the theory that hemorrhoids are caused by vascular hyperplasia of the arteriovenous network within the anorectal submucosa.

In 1937, Milligan and Morgan [38] described their technique to perform surgical excision of hemorrhoids. The hemorrhoid is dissected out from the underlying anal sphincter, the vascular pedicle is ligated, and the mucosal defects are left open and allowed to granulate by secondary intention (Figure 3). Different instruments are available to perform excision of the hemorrhoidal tissue, including electrocautery, scissors, scalpel, laser, bipolar scissors, linear staplers, LigaSure (Valleylab, Tyco Health Care Group), or Harmonic Scalpel (Ethicon Endo-Surgery, Inc.).

Ferguson's (closed) hemorrhoidectomy was developed in 1952 in the United States [39]. After excision of each hemorrhoid component, the ensuing defect is closed primarily.

Sir Alan Parks [40] in 1956 described a technique that dissects the submucosa containing the hemorrhoidal tissue with transfixation of the uppermost part of the pedicle. Reconstruction of the anal mucosa is done by fixing the mucosal flaps down to cover the wound, incorporating a largish bundle of internal sphincter. An area is deliberately left bare between the pedicle ligature and the mucosal fixation stitch.

Whitehead's hemorrhoidectomy, described by Whitehead [41] in 1882, was devised to eradicate enlarged internal hemorrhoidal tissue in a circumferential fashion and to relocate the prolapse dentate line, which often is a component of prolapsing hemorrhoids. At present, this procedure is rarely performed because of high complication rates, including stricture, loss of anal sensation, and development of mucosal ectropion [42].

Doppler-guided hemorrhoidal artery ligation was first described in 1995 by Morinaga et al. [43]. It is performed using a specially-designed proctoscope with an inbuilt Doppler probe that can locate feeding arteries; these vessels are then ligated using absorbable sutures. Disrupting the inflow to the vascular cushion is thought to reduce the size of the hemorrhoid.

Longo [44] recently proposed the use of a circular stapler instrument to perform hemorrhoidopexy. Thompson [45] suggested that the nature of hemorrhoids is the weakening and fragmentation of the tissue supporting the hemorrhoidal cushions, due to ageing and repeated passage of hard stool, leading to their descent and prolapse. The technique aims at reducing the hemorrhoidal prolapse and transecting the superior hemorrhoidal arteries.

A)

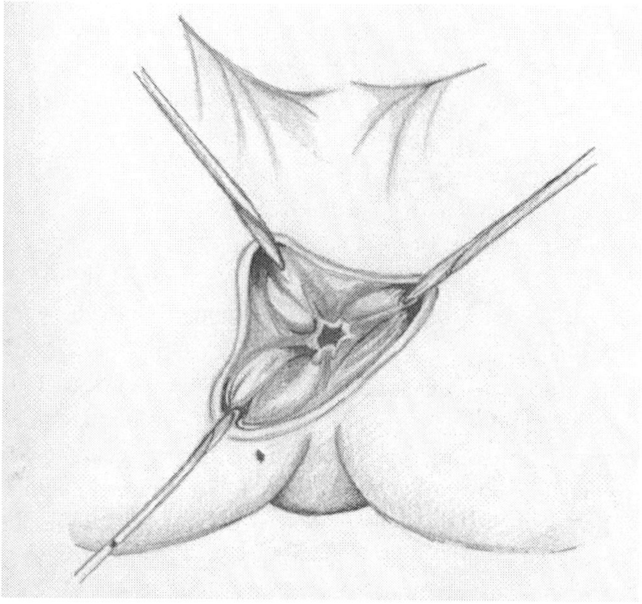

B)

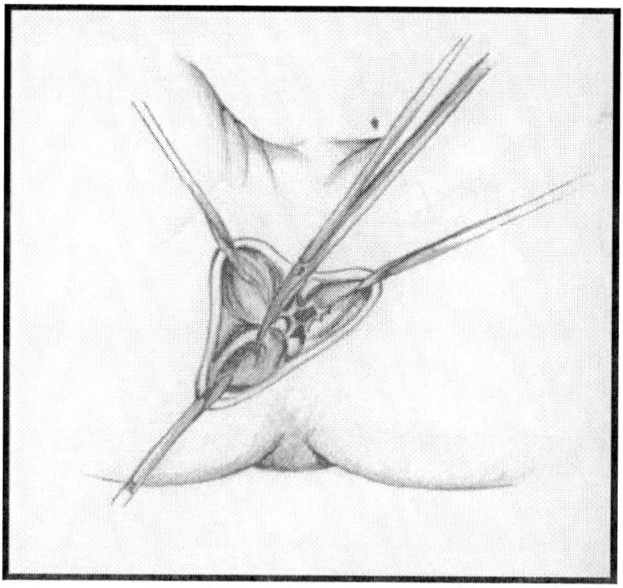

Figure 3. (Continued)

C)

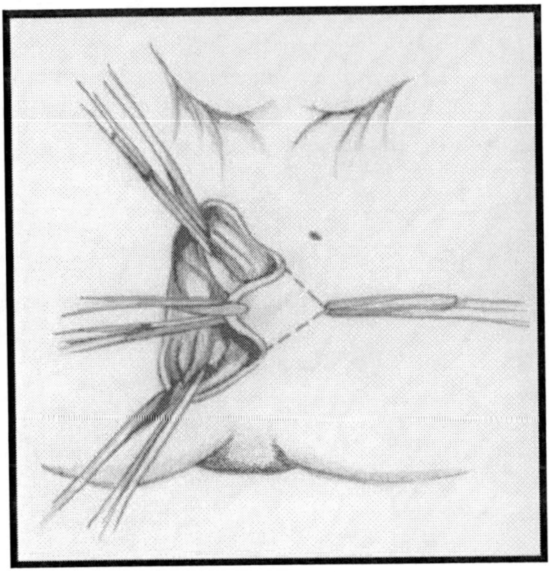

D)

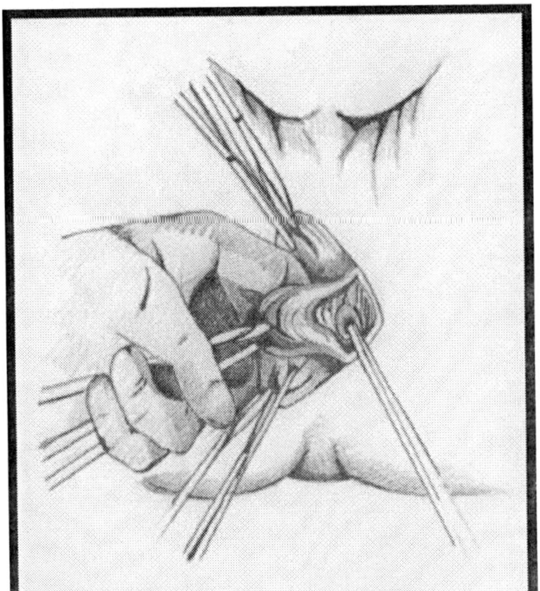

Figure 3. (Continued)

E)

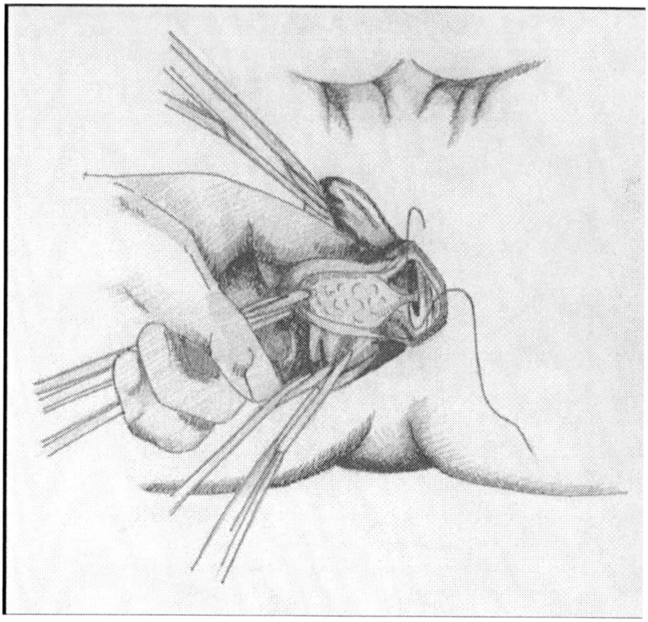

F)

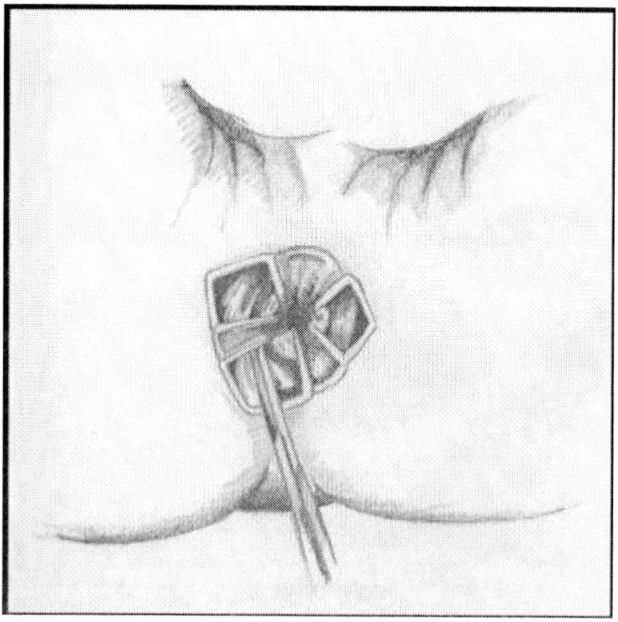

Figure 3. (Continued)

G)

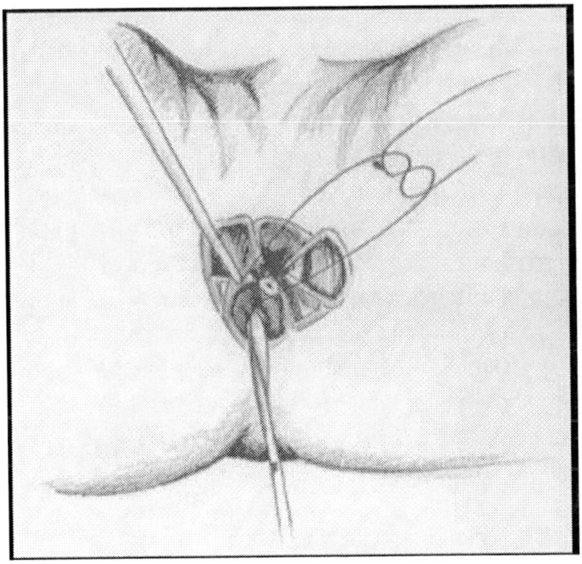

Figure 3. Milligan-Morgan procedure.

A) The patient is laid in the lithotomy position. Pean forceps are clipped on the base of each hemorrhoid and the pile is pulled out gently to expose the apex.

B) A second forceps is clipped at the level of the apex. This produces a triangular shape, called "triangle of exposure," which marks out the shape of the tissue to be cut.

C) A "V" shaped incision of the skin is made at the wide base of the hemorrhoid.

D) The hemorrhoidal tissue is dissected from the underlying sphincter muscle.

E) The excision of the hemorrhoid mass is completed by first ligating the pedicle.

F) At the end of the dissection, three triangular-shaped wounds are created with a wide base of approximately 1.0 cm. Dissection under the mucocutaneous bridges is performed to search for residual hemorrhoids.

G) The residual hemorrhoids are excised by first ligating the pedicle.

Hemorrhoidal prolapse is resolved by repositioning the hemorrhoidal masses into the anal canal and by reducing the venous engorgement with transection of the feeding arteries and redundant mucosa. This technique results in a stapled mucosa anastomosis in the rectum, at least 3 cm above the dentate line, where sensitive receptors are few. Moreover, any dissection or trauma in the area of anal mucosa and anoderm is avoided (Figure 4).

Ligation-anopexy (a fixation of the mucosa and submucosa of the hemorrhoidal region to the underlying internal sphincter) and open hemorrhoidopexy without the use of stapler (fixation of the anal mucosa to the rectal wall with four Z-stitches after removal of a small rectal mucosa flap about 4 cm from the dentate line) were recently described [46,47]. However, the preliminary results of these new techniques need to be confirmed on a larger number of patients, with a longer follow-up and comparisons with other established treatments.

A)

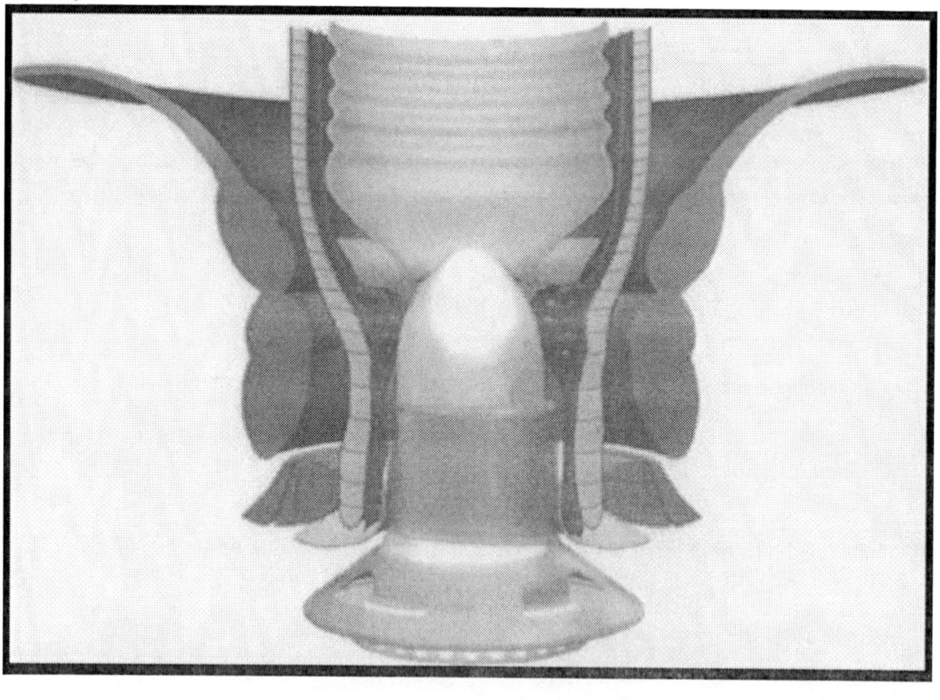

Figure 4. (Continued)

B)

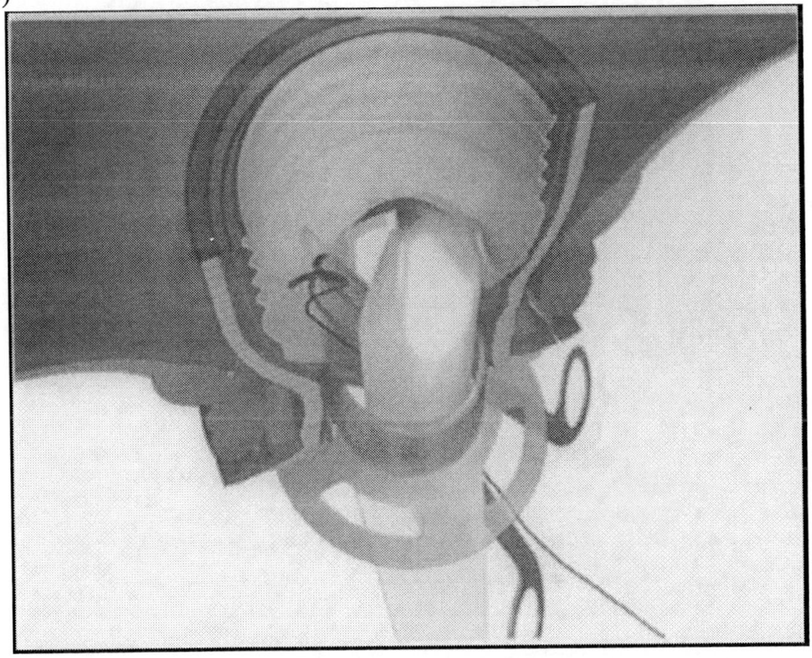

C)

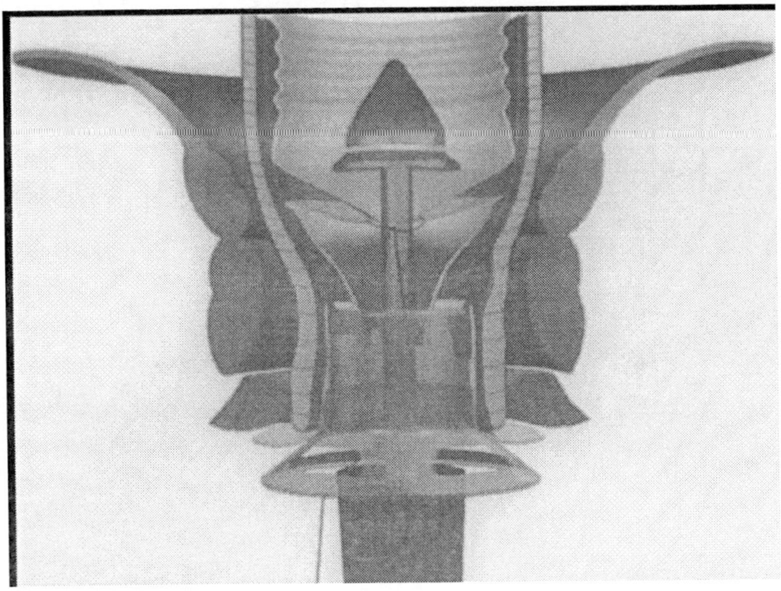

Figure 4. (Continued)

D)

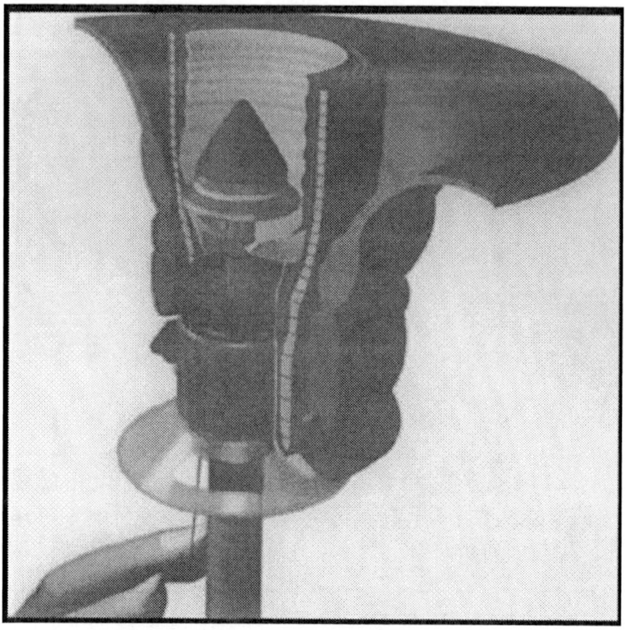

E)

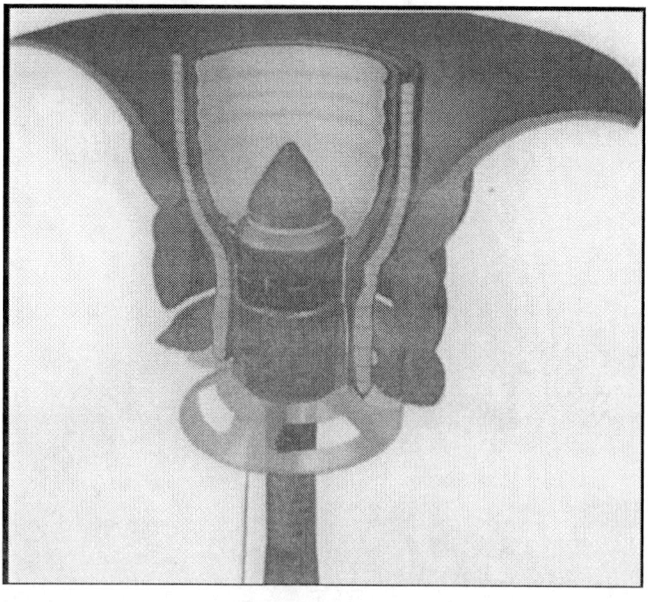

Figure 4. (Continued)

F)

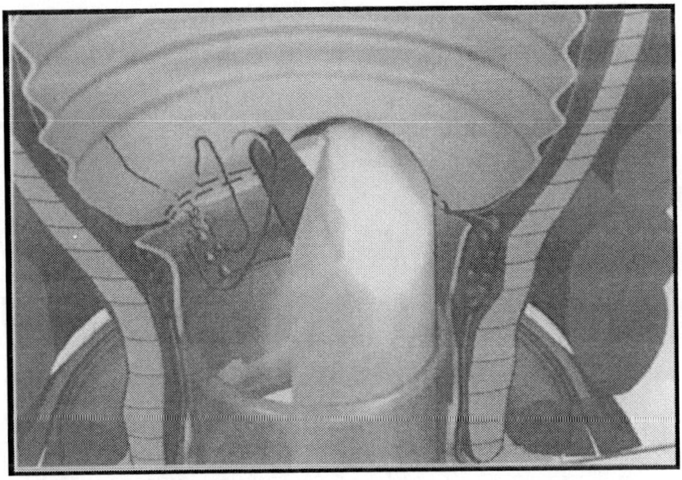

Figure 4. Stapled hemorrhoidopexy.

A) The patient is laid in the lithotomy position. The introduction of the circular anal dilator and the obturator causes the reduction of the prolapse of the anal skin and parts of the anal mucous membrane.

B) The obturator is removed and the purse-string suture anoscope is introduced through the dilator. By rotating the anoscope, it is possible to complete a purse-string suture around the entire anal circumference. The purse-string suture should be placed about 5 cm above the dentate line. The anoscope is withdrawn and the stapling device introduced with the anvil fully extended.

C) The purse-string suture is tightened. Both tails of the purse-string suture are pulled through the lateral ports of the stapler with the aid of the suture grasper.

D) With moderate traction on the purse-string, a simple maneuver draws the prolapsed mucous membrane into the casing of the circular stapling device.

E) The instrument is then tightened and held closed for 30 seconds to aid hemostasis. Firing the stapler releases a double staggered row of titanium staples through the tissue. A circular knife excises the redundant tissue. A circumferential column of mucosa is removed from the lower rectum.

F) The staple line, which should be positioned 3 cm above the dentate line, is inspected with the aid of the purse-string suture anoscope. Any bleeding point should be carefully oversewn.

COMPLICATIONS

Pain after surgery for hemorrhoids is a major worry. In order to reduce postoperative pain, various excision techniques have been proposed. Chung et al. [48] conducted a prospective double-blind study comparing different excision techniques: Harmonic Scalpel hemorrhoidectomy, bipolar scissors hemorrhoidectomy and regular scissors. The study showed that the Harmonic Scalpel was superior to the other methods in terms of postoperative pain and, consequently, patient satisfaction. LigaSure was associated with less postoperative pain when compared with Harmonic Scalpel in one randomized controlled trail [49]. In a recent review of the literature, LigaSure technique resulted in significantly less immediate postoperative pain after hemoroidectomy with respect to conventional diathermy techniques [50]. However, the added cost when performing the procedure with the LigaSure should be considered. A recent meta-analysis did not demonstrate any difference in pain scores with regard to open and closed hemorrhoidectomy [51]. Other surgical strategies to reduce pain have been introduced, such as limiting the incision [52], suturing only the vascular pedicle without an incision [53], and using a lateral internal sphincterotomy in conjunction with an external hemorrhoidectomy [54]. However, each strategy has had limited or mixed results. Proponents of hemorrhoidopexy with the use of circular staplers claim a reduction in postoperative pain and faster recovery compared to conventional excision procedures. A recent meta-analysis confirmed both of these advantages [55]. Metronidazole administration was found to be effective in reducing postoperative pain [56,57]. Local anesthetic infiltration after induction of anesthesia and before the surgical incision contributes to improvement in pain control after hemorrhoidectomy [58]. Topical diltiazem showed marginal benefit in reducing pain after surgery [59]. Glyceryl trinitrate ointment improved wound healing with conflicting results with respect to postoperative pain reduction [60,61]. Injected butulinum showed superior efficacy compared to glyceryl trinitrate ointment [62]. Topical sucralfate cream can both reduce pain and improve wound healing after open hemorrhoidectomy [63]. Regardless of the above mentioned methods used, effective postoperative pain management is required. Ketorolac has demonstrated considerable efficacy in managing posthemorrhoidectomy pain [64]. The use of stool softeners can help avoid straining and reduce the pain at the first postoperative bowel movement. Starting this four days before surgery may be beneficial [65]. The avoidance of bulky packs and dressings in the anal canal is also known to reduce postsurgical pain [66].

Postoperative hemorrhage is a relatively common complication. Bleeding in the immediate postoperative period is almost always due to inadequate intraoperative hemostasis. In the existing literature, this complication occurs in 4% to 25% of cases [67-76]. Bleeding predominantly affects patients with fourth-degree hemorrhoids [75,76]. Most bleeding complications occur during operation at the staple line and should be managed with suture of the bleeding points, after a careful inspection of the stapled suture line [75,76]. After the introduction of the newer circular stapler (PPH03, Ethicon Endo-Surgery, Cincinnati, OH), which has a closed staple height of 0.75 mm, bleeding after stapled hemorrhoidopexy may be reduced because of an increase in compression on rectal tissue and blood vessels. A significant reduction of intraoperative bleeding with the use of PPH03 compared with PPH01 (Ethicon Endo-Surgery, Cincinnati, OH) was reported in a recent randomized trial [77].

Another common complication after surgery for hemorrhoids is acute retention of urine. After conventional open hemorrhoidectomy, the estimated incidence of urinary retention ranges from 0% to 34% and from 0% to 22% after stapled hemorrhoidopexy [78,79]. In a meta-analysis comparing stapled hemorrhoidopexy and open hemorrhoidectomy, incidence of urinary retention was similar [80]. The expected reduction of postoperative urinary retention after stapled hemorrhoidopexy, caused by less postoperative pain, was not confirmed in the study by Senagore et al. [81], which showed that pain was not a risk factor for urinary retention.

Sepsis after surgery for hemorrhoids is uncommon, but it may be catastrophic. Cases of serious sepsis after both conventional and stapled hemorrhoidectomy were reported [82,84]. Guidelines do not exist for prophylactic antibiotics for hemorrhoid surgery. However, we recommend routine use of prophylactic antibiotic therapy to avoid these life-threatening complications.

Anal stenosis is a narrowing of the anal canal. This narrowing may result from a true anatomic stricture or a muscular and functional stenosis. The main cause of anal stenosis is caused by overzealous hemorrhoidectomy. Removal of large areas of anoderm and hemorrhoidal rectal mucosa, without sparing of adequate muco-cutaneous bridges, leads to scarring and a progressive chronic stricture. After conventional procedures, the incidence of anal stenosis is 0–6% [16]. Stenoses caused by stapled hemorrhoidopexy are presumably rectal stenoses, since the causing event was a resection of rectal mucosa. One potential mechanism that might cause stenosis is ring dehiscence followed by submucous inflammation. Another theoretical cause is that the stapled ring is placed too deep in the anal canal and that the squamous skin cells react by scarring and shrinking. In a large study anal stenosis was observed in only 0.8% of cases [85].

Control of defecation involves a complex interaction of various factors. After hemorrhoid surgery incontinence may result from sphincter lesions, loss of sensitive anoderm and loss of reservoir (rectal resection, reduced rectal compliance due to rectal resection). Continence disorders following hemorrhoidectomy are reported to vary between 0% and 20% [86]. The type of procedure used and the surgical expertise are important factors influencing the occurrence of these complications. The upper replacement instead of excision of the piles, carried out by stapled hemorrhoidopexy, should reduce postoperative incontinence, as hemorrhoids are important factors of anal continence [87]. However, postoperative incontinence after stapled hemorrhoidectomy was reported in up to 28% of cases [86]. In most patients incontinence is transitory, due to excessive anal stretching secondary to circular anal dilator insertion [87]. At long-term follow-up, persistent continence problems were reported in a minority of patients with no significant difference with respect to conventional hemorrhoidectomy [88-91].

Tenesmus, frequency and faecal urgency are variably associated with hemorrhoid surgery and are usually transient and self-limiting.

RESULTS

Traditionally, hemorrhoid surgery was considered a painful operation, and pain is still the main concern of patients undergoing surgery. Stapled hemorrhoidopexy was recommended because of the short operative time, slight postoperative pain, and faster recovery. The advantages of this procedure were confirmed by a recent systematic review of randomized trials comparing stapled and conventional hemorrhoidectomy [55]. However, in the recent literature, a significant incidence of recurrence after stapled hemorrhoidopexy was reported. In studies evaluating stapled hemorrhoidopexy and conventional hemorrhoidectomy for grade III and grade IV hemorrhoids with an adequate and systematic follow-up (>1 year), the incidence of recurrence was 0% to 26% and 0% to 10.8%, respectively; reoperation rate was up to 16.7% after stapled hemorrhoidopexy [69,72,88-94]. After conventional Ferguson's hemorrhoidectomy, a redo surgery for recurrent hemorrhoids was necessary in 0.8% of cases in a large series [95]. In a study with a minimum follow-up of five years, recurrence occurred in 18.2% of patients and reoperation was performed in 7.2% of cases after stapled hemorrhoidopexy [75]. However, when long-term control of hemorrhoid-related symptoms was considered, no significant difference was found between stapled hemorrhoidopexy and conventional hemorrhoidectomy with exception of the presence of prolapse [89]. In a large part of patients with recurrence after stapled hemorrhoidopexy symptoms related to hemorrhoids are absent or moderate [75]. These data may explain why the higher incidence of recurrence after stapled hemorrhoidopexy does not affect the long-term results in terms of patient satisfaction. Long-term satisfaction with the Milligan–Morgan procedure was achieved in 67% of patients in a large retrospective multicenter study [96]. After stapled hemorrhoidopexy patients satisfaction was up to 89.7% [75]. Recurrence rate, reintervention, and complications are important outcome measures when assessing a procedure; however, quality of life and patient satisfaction are also important and need to be considered. A very recent study assessed quality of life, patients' satisfaction and patients' approval of the procedure and their willingness for a repeat procedure. The authors concluded that when compared with conventional hemorrhoidectomy stapled hemorrhoidopexy is favored by the patients [97].

According to some authors, recurrent rectal prolapse was significantly more frequent in patients with fourth-degree hemorrhoids, so that they may not represent an appropriate indication for stapled hemorrhoidopexy [75,76,98]. This may be related to the increased probability of incomplete mucosal resection in Grade IV hemorrhoids, which may occur when the volume of prolapsed tissue exceeds the volume of the stapler casing. Double stapling, according to the stapled transanal rectal resection proposed by Longo [99] to treat obstructive defecation syndrome, allows to achieve a more complete hemorrhoidopexy and may be appropriate for grade IV hemorrhoids [100].

Repeated stapled hemorrhoidopexy can by performed safely and with satisfactory results in patients with recurrent hemorrhoids [101].

Conclusion

Currently, there is a variety of surgical procedures that are available to treat hemorrhoids, and most have similar success rates. Stapled hemorrhoidopexy has gained vast popularity, mainly because of reduced postoperative pain with respect to conventional hemorrhoidectomy. However, at present the main issue with this technique is its durability. In particular, the high incidence of recurrence, especially in fourth-degree hemorrhoids, casts serious doubt regarding its efficacy with respect to conventional hemorrhoidectomy. Stapled transanal rectal resection may be an alternative to simple stapled hemorrhoidopexy in fourth-degree hemorrhoids, whenever the circumference of the hemorrhoidal prolapse exceeds the circumference of the stapler case and/or internal mucosal prolapse is detected after the introduction of the anal retractor. Further prospective studies are necessary to evaluate this new approach.

We believe that the surgeon should discuss with the patients the advantages and drawbacks of each surgical procedure and let the patient choose whether to accept a higher recurrence rate to take advantage of the short-term benefits of stapled hemorrhoidopexy.

Acknowledgments

We thank Mrs. Rita Massimi for the drawings included in Figures 1 and 3.

References

[1] Haas PA, Haas GP, Schmaltz S, Fox TA Jr. The prevalence of hemorrhoids. *Dis. Colon. Rectum* 1983;26:435–9.

[2] Bennett WG, Cerda JJ. Dietary fiber: fact and fiction. *Dig. Dis.* 1996;14:43–58.

[3] Spiller RC. Pharmacology of dietary fiber. *Pharmacol. Ther.* 1994;62:407–27.

[4] Alonso-Coello P, Mills E, Heels-Ansdell D, Lopez-Yarto M, Zhou Q, Johanson JF, Guyatt G. Fiber for the treatment of hemorrhoid complications: a systematic review and meta-analysis. *Am. J. Gastroenterol.* 2006;101:181-8.

[5] Pigot F, Siproudhis L, Allaert FA. Risk factors associated with hemorrhoidal symptoms in specialized consultation. *Gastroenterol. Clin. Biol.* 2005;29:1270-4.

[6] Alonso-Coello P, Zhou Q, Martinez-Zapata MJ, Mills E, Heels-Ansdell D, Johanson JF, Guyatt G. Meta-analysis of flavonoids for the treatment of haemorrhoids. *Br. J. Surg.* 2006;93(8):909-20.

[7] Menteş BB, Görgül A, Tatlicioğlu E, Ayoğlu F, Unal S. Efficacy of calcium dobesilate in treating acute attacks of hemorrhoidal disease. *Dis. Colon. Rectum 2001*;44:1489-95.

[8] Acheson AG, Scholefield JH. Management of haemorrhoids. *BMJ* 2008;336:380-3.

[9] Tjandra JJ, Tan JJ, Lim JF, Murray-Green C, Kennedy ML, Lubowski DZ. Rectogesic (glyceryl trinitrate 0.2%) ointment relieves symptoms of

haemorrhoids associated with high resting anal canal pressures. *Colorectal. Dis.* 2007;9:457-63.

[10] Karanlik H, Akturk R, Camlica H, Asoglu O. The effect of glyceryl trinitrate ointment on posthemorrhoidectomy pain and wound healing: results of a randomized, double-blind, placebo-controlled study. *Dis. Colon. Rectum.* 2009;52:280-5.

[11] Guy RJ, Seow-Choen F. Septic complications after treatment of haemorrhoids. *Br. J. Surg.* 2003;90:147-56.

[12] Senapati A, Nicholls RJ. A randomised trial to compare the results of injection sclerotherapy with a bulk laxative alone in the treatment of bleeding haemorrhoids. *Int. J. Colorectal. Dis.* 1988;3:124-6.

[13] Takano M, Iwadare J, Ohba H, Takamura H, Masuda Y, Matsuo K, Kanai T, Ieda H, Hattori Y, Kurata S, Koganezawa S, Hamano K, Tsuchiya S. Sclerosing therapy of internal hemorrhoids with a novel sclerosing agent. Comparison with ligation and excision. *Int. J. Colorectal. Dis.* 2006; 21:44-51.

[14] Walker AJ, Leicester RJ, Nicholls RJ, Mann CV. A prospective study of infrared coagulation, injection and rubber band ligation in the treatment of haemorrhoids. *Int. J. Colorectal. Dis.* 1990;5:113-6.

[15] Dennison A, Whiston RJ, Rooney S, Chadderton RD, Wherry DC, Morris DL. A randomized comparison of infrared photocoagulation with bipolar diathermy for the outpatient treatment of hemorrhoids. *Dis. Colon. Rectum.* 1990;33:32–4.

[16] American Gastroenterological Association. Technical review on the diagnosis and treatment of hemorrhoids. *Gastroenterology* 2004;126:1463-73.

[17] Wright R, Kruz K, Kirby S. A prospective crossover trial of direct current electrotherapy in symptomatic hemorrhoidal disease. *Gastrointest. Endosc.* 1991;37:621-3.

[18] Salvati EP. Nonoperative management of hemorrhoids. Evolution of the office management of hemorrhoids. *Dis. Colon. Rectum.* 1999; 42:989-93.

[19] Blaisdell PC. Prevention of massive hemorrhage secondary to hemorrhoidectomy. *Surg. Gynecol. Obstet.*1958;106:485-8.

[20] Barron J. Office ligation treatment of hemorrhoids. *Dis. Colon. Rectum.* 1963;6:109-13.

[21] Trowers EA, Ganga U, Rizk R, Ojo E, Hodges D. Endoscopic hemorrhoidal ligation: preliminary clinical experience. *Gastrointest. Endosc.* 1998;48:49-52.

[22] Wrobleski DE, Corman ML, Veidenheimer MC, Coller JA. Long-term evaluation of rubber ring ligation in hemorrhoidal disease. *Dis. Colon. Rectum.* 1980;23:478–82.

[23] Steinberg DM, Liegois H, Alexander-Williams J. Long term review of the results of rubber band ligation of haemorrhoids. *Br. J. Surg.* 1975;62:144–6.

[24] Savioz D, Roche B, Glauser T, Dobrinov A, Ludwig C, Marti MC. Rubber band ligation of hemorrhoids: relapse as a function of time. *Int. J. Colorectal. Dis.* 1998;13:154-6.

[25] Walker AJ, Leicester RJ, Nicholls RJ, Mann CV. A prospective study of infrared coagulation, injection and rubber band ligation in the treatment of haemorrhoids. *Int .J. Colorectal. Dis.* 1990;5:113-6.

[26] Wechter DG, Luna GK. An unusual complication of rubber band ligation of hemorrhoids. *Dis. Colon. Rectum.* 1987;30:137-40.

[27] Johanson JF, Rimm A. Optimal nonsurgical treatment of hemorrhoids: a comparative analysis of infrared coagulation, rubber band ligation, and injection sclerotherapy. *Am. J. Gastroenterol.* 1992;87:1600–6.

[28] MacRae HM, Temple LK, McLeod RS. A meta-analysis of hemorrhoidal treatments. *Semin. C R Surg.* 2002;13:77–83.

[29] Shanmugam V, Thaha MA, Rabindranath KS, Campbell KL, Steele RJ, Loudon MA. Systematic review of randomized trials comparing rubber band ligation with excisional haemorrhoidectomy. *Br. J. Surg.* 2005; 92:1481-7.

[30] Chew SS, Marshall L, Kalish L, Tham J, Grieve DA, Douglas PR, Newstead GL. Short-term and long-term results of combined sclerotherapy and rubber band ligation of hemorrhoids and mucosal prolapse. *Dis. Colon. Rectum.* 2003;46:1232–7.

[31] Wolkomir AF, Luchtefeld MA. Surgery for symptomatic hemorrhoids and anal fissure in Crohn's disease. *Dis. Colon. Rectum.* 1993; 36:545-7.

[32] Lord PH. A new regimen for the treatment of haemorrhoids. *Proc. R. Soc. Med* 1968;61:935-6.

[33] De Roover DM, Hoofwijk AG, Van Vroonhoven TJ. Lateral internal sphincterotomy in the treatment of four degree hemorrhoids. *Br. J. Surg. 1989*; 76:1181.

[34] Deutsch AA, Moshkovitz M, Nudelman I, Dinari G, Reiss R. Anal pressure measurements in the study of hemorrhoid etiology and their relation to treatment. *Dis. Colon. Rectum.* 1987;30:855–7.

[35] McIntyre IM, Balfour TW. Results of the Lord non operative treatment for haemorrhoids. *Lancet* 1972;1:1094-5.

[36] Snooks S, Henry MM, Swash M. Faecal incontinence after anal dilatation. *B.r J. Surg.* 1984;71:617-8.

[37] Pescatori M, Favetta U, Navarra L. Anal pressures after hemorrhoidectomy. *Int. J. Colorectal Dis.* 1998;13:149.

[38] Milligan ETC, Morgan CN, Jones LE, Officer R. Surgical Anatomy of the Anal Canal and Operative Treatment of Haemorrohids. Lancet 1937;2:1119-24.

[39] Ferguson JA, Mazier WP, Ganchrow MI, Friend WG. The closed technique of hemorrhoidectomy. *Surgery* 1971;70:480–4.

[40] Parks AG. The surgical treatment of haemorrhoids. *Br. J. Surg.* 1956;43:337-51.

[41] Whitehead W. Surgical treatment of haemorrhoids. *Br. Med. J.* 1982;1:148-50.

[42] Hemorrhoids. In: Corman ML, ed. Colon and rectal surgery. 5th ed. Philadelphia: Lippincott Williams and Wilkins; 2004:177–253.

[43] Morinaga K, Hasuda K, Ikeda T. A novel therapy for internal hemorrhoids: ligation of the hemorrhoidal artery with a newly devised instrument (Moricorn) in conjunction with a Doppler flowmeter. *Am. J. Gastroenterol.* 1995;90:610-3.

[44] Longo A. Treatment of haemorrhoids disease by reduction of mucosa and haemorrhoidal prolapse with a circular suturing device: a new procedure. Proceedings of the 6th World Congress of Endoscopic Surgery, Rome, Italy, June 3–6, 1998.

[45] Thomson WH. The nature of haemorrhoids. *Br. J. Surg.* 1975;62:542-52.

[46] Hussein HM. Ligation anopexy for treatment of advanced hemorrhoidal disease. *Dis. Colon. Rectum.* 2001;44:1887-90.

[47] Pakravan F, Helmes C, Baeten, C. Transanal open hemorrhoidopexy. *Dis. Colon. Rectum.* 2009; 52:503-6.

[48] Chung CC, Ha JP, Tai YP, Tsang WW, Li MK. Double-blind, randomized trial comparing Harmonic Scalpel hemorrhoidectomy, bipolar scissors hemorrhoidectomy, and scissors excision: ligation technique. *Dis. Colon. Rectum.* 2002;45:789–94.

[49] Kwok SY, Chung CC, Tsui KK, Li MK. A double-blind, randomized trial comparing LigaSure and Harmonic Scalpel hemorrhoidectomy. *Dis. Colon. Rectum.* 2005;48:344–8.

[50] Nienhuijs S, de Hingh I. Conventional versus LigaSure hemorrhoidectomy for patients with symptomatic hemorrhoids. *Cochrane Database of Systematic Reviews* 2009, Issue 1.

[51] Ho YH, Buettner PG. Open compared with closed haemorrhoidectomy: meta-analysis of randomized controlled trials. *Tech. Coloproctol.* 2007; 11:135–43.

[52] Ui Y. Anoderm-preserving, completely closed hemorrhoidectomy with no mucosal incision. *Dis Colon Rectum* 1997;40:S99–S101.

[53] Patel N, O'Connor T. Suture haemorrhoidectomy: a day-only alternative. *Aust. N. Z. J. Surg.* 1996;66:830–1.

[54] Mathai V, Ong BC, Ho YH. Randomized controlled trial of lateral internal sphincterotomy with haemorrhoidectomy. *Br. J. Surg.* 1996;83:380–2.

[55] Shao WJ, Li GC, Zhang ZH, Yang BL, Sun GD, Chen YQ. Systematic review and meta-analysis of randomized controlled trials comparing stapled haemorrhoidopexy with conventional haemorrhoidectomy. *Br. J. Surg.* 2008;95:147-60.

[56] Carapeti EA, Kamm MA, McDonald PJ, Philips RKS. Double-blind randomised controlled trial of effect of metronidazole on pain after daycase haemorrhoidectomy. *Lancet* 1998;351:169–72.

[57] Ala S, Saeedi M, Eshghi F, Mirzabeygi P. Topical metronidazole can reduce pain after surgery and pain on defecation in postoperative hemorrhoidectomy. *Dis. Colon. Rectum* .2008;51:235-8.

[58] Vinson-Bonnet B, Coltat JC, Fingerhut A, Bonnet F. Local infiltration with ropivacaine improves immediate postoperative pain control after hemorrhoidal surgery. *Dis. Colon. Rectum.* 2002;45:104-8.

[59] Silverman R, Bendick PJ, Wasvary HJ. A randomized, prospective, double-blind, placebo-controlled trial of the effect of a calcium channel blocker ointment on pain after hemorrhoidectomy. *Dis. Colon. Rectum.* 2005; 48:1913-6.

[60] Tan KY, Sng KK, Tay KH, Lai JH, Eu KW. Randomized clinical trial of 0·2 per cent glyceryl trinitrate ointment for wound healing and pain reduction after open diathermy haemorrhoidectomy. *Br. J. Sur.* 2006;93: 1464–8.

[61] Karanlik H, Akturk R, Camlica H, Asoglu O. The effect of glyceryl trinitrate ointment on posthemorrhoidectomy pain and wound healing: results of a randomized, double-blind, placebo-controlled study. *Dis. Colon. Rectum* .2009;52:280-5.

[62] Patti R, Almasio PL, Arcara M, Sammartano S, Romano P, Fede C, Di Vita G. Botulinum toxin vs topical glyceryl trinitrate ointment for pain control in patients undergoing hemorrhoidectomy: a randomized trial. *Dis. Colon. Rectum.* 2006;49:1741-8.

[63] Gupta PJ, Heda PS, Kalaskar S, Tamaskar VP. Topical sucralfate decreases pain after hemorrhoidectomy and improves healing: a randomized, blinded, controlled study. *Dis Colon Rectum* 2008;51:231-4.

[64] O'Donovan S, Ferrara A, Larach S, Williamson P. Intraoperative use of Toradol facilitates outpatient hemorrhoidectomy. *Dis. Colon. Rectum.* 1994;34:793-9.

[65] London NJ, Bramley PD, Windle R. Effect of four days of preoperative lactulose on posthaemorrhoidectomy pain: Results of a placebo-controlled trial. *Br. Med. J.* 1987;295:363-4.

[66] Ingram M, Wright TA, Ingoldby CJ. A prospective randomized study of calcium alginate (Sorbsan) versus standard gauze packing following haemorrhoidectomy. *J R Coll Surg. Edinb.*1998;43:308-9.

[67] Chen HH, Wang JY, Changchien CR, Chen JS, Hsu KC, Chiang JM, Yeh CY, Tang R. Risk factors associated with posthemorrhoidectomy secondary hemorrhage. *Dis. Colon. Rectum.* 2002;45:1096-9.

[68] Bleday R, Pena JP, Rothenberger DA, Goldberg SM, Buls JG. Symptomatic hemorrhoids: current incidence of complications of operative therapy. *Dis. Colo.n Rectum* 1992;35:477-81.

[69] Boccasanta P, Capretti PG, Venturi M, Cioffi U, De Simone M, Salamina G, Contessini-Avesani E, Peracchia A. Randomized controlled trial between stapled circumferential mucosectomy and conventional circular hemorrhoidectomy in advanced hemorrhoids with external mucosal prolapsed. *Am. J. Surg.* 2001;182:64-8.

[70] Mehigan BJ, Monson JRT, Hartley JE. Stapling procedure for haemorrhoids versus Milligan-Morgan haemorrhoidectomy: randomized controlled trial. *Lancet* 2000;355:782-5.

[71] Ho YH, Cheong WK, Tsang C, Ho J, Eu KW, Tang CL, Seow-Choen F. Stapled hemorrhoidectomy– cost and effectiveness. Randomized, controlled trial including incontinence scoring, anorectal manometry and endoanal ultrasound assessment at up to three months. *Dis. Colon. Rectum.* 2000;46: 1666-75.

[72] Ganio E, Altomare DF, Gabrielli F, Milito G, Canuti S. Prospective randomized multi center trial comparing stapled with open hemorrhoidectomy. *B.r J. Surg.* 2001;88:669-74.

[73] Palimento D, Picchio M, Attanasio U, Lombardi A, Bambini C, Renda A. Stapled and open hemorrhoidectomy: randomized controller trial of early results. *World J. Surg.* 2003;27:203-7.

[74] Ng KH, Ho KS, Ooi BS, Tang CL, Eu KW. Experience of 3711 stapled haemorrhoidectomy operations. *Br. J. Surg.* 2006;93:226-30.

[75] Ceci F, Picchio M, Palimento D, Calì B, Corelli S, Spaziani E. Long-term outcome of stapled hemorrhoidopexy for Grade III and Grade IV hemorrhoids. *Dis. Colon. Rectum.* 2008;51:1107-12.

[76] Finco C, Sarzo G, Savastano S, Degregori S, Merigliano S. Stapled haemorrhoidectomy in fourth degree haemorrhoidal prolapse: is it worthwhile? *Colorectal. Dis.* 2006;8:130-4.

[77] Arroyo A, Perez-Vicente F, Miranda E, Sánchez A, Serrano P, Candela F, Oliver I, Calpena R. Prospective randomized clinical trial comparing two different circular staplers for mucosectomy in the treatment of hemorrhoids. *World. J. Surg.* 2006;30:1305–10.

[78] Zaheer S, Reilly WT, Pemberton JH, Ilstrup D. Urinary retention after operations for benign anorectal diseases. *Dis. Colon. Rectum.* 1998;41:696-704.

[79] Wilson MS, Pope V, Doran HE, Fearn SJ, Brough WA. Objective comparison of stapled anopexy and open hemorrhoidectomy. *Dis. Colon. Rectum* 2002;45:1437-44.

[80] Lan P, Wu X, Zhou X, Wang J, Zhang L. The safety and efficacy of stapled hemorrhoidectomy in the treatment of hemorrhoids: a systemic review and meta-analysis of the randomized controlled trials. *Int. J. Colorectal. Dis.* 2006;21:172-8.

[81] Senagore AJ, Singer M, Abcarian H, Fleshman J, Corman M, Wexner S, Nivatvongs S; Procedure for Prolapse and Hemmorrhoids (PPH) Multicenter Study Group. A prospective, randomized, controlled, multicenter trial comparing stapled hemorrhoidopexy and Ferguson hemorrhoidectomy: perioperative and one-year results. *Dis. Colon. Rectum.* 2004;47:1824-36.

[82] Basoglu M, Gul O, Yildirgan I, Balik AA, Ozbey I, Oren D. Fournier's gangrene: review of fifteen cases. *Am. Surg.* 1997;63:1019-21.

[83] Molloy RG, Kingsmore D. Life threatening pelvic sepsis after stapled haemorrhoidectomy. *Lancet* 2000; 355: 810.

[84] Cirocco CW. Life threatening sepsis and mortality following stapled hemorrhoidopexy *Surgery* 2008;143:824-9.

[85] Ravo B, Amato A, Bianco V, Boccasanta P, Bottini C, Carriero A, Milito G, Dodi G, Mascagni D, Orsini S, Pietroletti R, Ripetti V, Tagariello GB. Complications after stapled hemorrhoidectomy: can they be prevented? *Tech. Coloproctol.* 2002;6:83-8.

[86] Thekkinkattil DK, Dunham RJ, O'Herlihy S, Finan PJ, Sagar PM, Burke DA. Measurement of anal cushions in idiopathic faecal incontinence. *Br. J. Surg* .2009;96:680-4.

[87] Ho YH, Seow-Choen F, Tsang C, Eu KW. Randomized trial assessing anal sphincter injuries after stapled haemorrhoidectomy. *Br. J. Surg.* 2001;88: 1449-55.

[88] Ganio E, Altomare DF, Milito G, Gabrielli F, Canuti S. Long-term out come of a multicentre randomized clinical trial of stapled haemorrhoidopexy versus Milligan-Morgan haemorrhoidectomy. *Br. J. Sur.g* 2007;94:1033-7.

[89] Smyth EF, Baker RP, Wilken BJ, Hartley JE, White TJ, Monson JR. Stapled versus excision haemorrhoidectomy: long-term follow-up of a randomized controlled trial. *Lancet* 2003;361:1437-8.

[90] Au-Yong I, Rowsell M, Hemingway DM. Randomized controlled clinical trial of stapled haemorrhoidectomy vs. conventional haemorrhoidectomy: a three and a half year follow-up. *Colorectal Dis.* 2004;6:37-8.

[91] Picchio M, Palimento D, Attanasio U, Renda A. Stapled vs. open hemorrhoidectomy: long-term outcome of a randomized controlled trial. *Int. J. Colorectal. Dis.* 2006;21:668-9.

[92] Racalbuto A, Aliotta I, Corsaro G, Lanteri R, Di Cataldo A, Licata A. Hemorrhoidal stapler prolapsectomy vs Milligan-Morgan hemorrhoid-ectomy: a long-term randomized trial. *Int. J. Colorecta.l Dis.* 2004;19:239-44.

[93] Kairaluoma M, Nuorva K, Kellokumpu I. Day-case stapled (circular) vs diathermy hemorrhoidectomy: a randomized controlled trial evaluating surgical and functional outcome. *Dis. Colon. Rectum.* 2003;46:93-9.

[94] Ortiz H, Marzo J, Armendariz P. Randomized trial of stapled haemorrhoidopexy versus conventional diathermy haemorrhoidectomy. *Br. J. Surg.* 2002;89:1376–81.

[95] Guenin MO, Rosenthal R, Kern B, Peterli R, von Flüe M, Ackermann C. Long-term results and patient satisfaction after Ferguson's hemor rhoidectomy. *Dis. Colon. Rectum.* 2005;48:1523-7.

[96] Johannsson HO, Graf W, Pahlman L. Long-term results of haemor-rhoidectomy. *Eur. J. Surg.* 2002;168:485-9.

[97] Thaha MA, Campbell KL, Kazmi SA, Irvine LA, Khalil A, Binnie NR, Hendry WS, Walker A, Staines HJ, Steele RJ. Prospective randomised multi-centre trial comparing the clinical efficacy, safety and patient acceptability of circular stapled anopexy with closed diathermy haemor-rhoidectomy. *Gut* 2009;58:668-78.

[98] Mattana C, Coco C, Manno A, Verbo A, Rizzo G, Petito L, Sermoneta D. Stapled hemorrhoidopexy and Milligan Morgan hemorrhoidectomy in the cure of fourth-degree hemorrhoids: long-term evaluation and clinical results. *Dis. Colon. Rectum.* 2007;50:1770-5.

[99] Longo A. Obstructed defecation because of rectal pathologies. Novel surgical treatment: stapled transanal resection (STARR). *Annual Cleveland Clinic Florida Colorectal Disease Symposium*, Fort Lauderdale, Florida, January 2005.

[100] Boccasanta P, Venturi M, Roviaro G. Stapled transanal rectal resection versus stapled anopexy in the cure of hemorrhoids associated with rectal prolapse. A randomized controlled trial. *Int. J. Colorectal. Dis.* 2007;22: 245-51.

[101] Raahave D, Jepsen LV, Pedersen IK. Primary and repeated stapled hemorrhoidopexy for prolapsing hemorrhoids: follow-up to five years. *Dis. Colon. Rectum.* 2008;51:334-41.

In: Hemorrhoids: Symptoms, Diagnosis...
Authors: P. Salinitri et al., pp. 55-78
ISBN: 978-1-60876-478-5

Chapter 3

STAPLED HAEMORRHOIDOPEXY: FROM PATHOLOGY TO CLINICAL OUTCOME AND REINTERVENTIONS

Pierpaolo Sileri[1], Stefano D'Ugo, Domenico Benavoli, Vito M. Stolfi, and Achille Gaspari

Departments of Surgery, University of Rome Tor Vergata, Rome Italy

ABSTRACT:

Stapled haemorrhoidopexy (SH) is an attractive alternative to conventional haemorrhoidectomy (CH) because of reduced postoperative pain, shorter hospital stay and earlier return to normal activities. Over the last decade, SH gained wide acceptance but this enthusiastic use has been tempered by increasing reports of specific technique related complications including occasional life threatening sepsis and deaths. Complications rate has been reported as high as 31%.

Data on patients undergoing haemorrhoidectomy at our unit or referred to us are prospectively entered in a database.

Patients and methods: We report our experience on 425 symptomatic patients who underwent haemorrhoidectomy at our Institution: 110 underwent SH while 315 underwent conventional haemorrhoidectomy with similar follow-up period (25±14 vs 32±16 months).

1 Corresponding author: Pierpaolo Sileri, MD, MS, PHD, Cattedra Chirurgia Generale, Policlinico Tor Vergata, 6B, Viale Oxford 81, 00133, Rome, Italy, Ph +393339137249; Fax +390620902927, Email:piersileri@yahoo.com.

Clinical outcome was assessed by a validated questionnaire on postoperative symptoms and satisfaction supplemented by the Wexner incontinence score. Data on bleeding, body temperature, pain after defecation, prolapse, incontinence, faecal urgency was prospectively recorded and analysed using Fisher exact and Mann-Whitney tests.

Results: Operating time between SH and CH was similar being 28.3±8.7 and 26±8.8 minutes respectively. Hospitalization rates were similar between SH and CH (2.7% vs 1.6%).

Likewise, no differences were observed in terms of ER admissions (7.3% vs 3.8%) and hospital readmissions (3.6% vs 2.2%) between SH and CH.

Overall early and late complication rates were similar between SH and CH.

Despite an increased quote of anal fissure, disabling chronic pain and recurrences were observed after SH when compared to CH, no significative differences were observed in terms of early and late complications between SH and CH (please refer to tables I and II).

Significant differences were observed in terms of pain (expressed as VAS) during the first postoperative week (please refer to figures 1 and 2). Patients who underwent CH experienced more severe pain (expressed as VAS score >7) than SH at 5, 6 and 7 postoperative day. We did not observed differences between SH and CH in terms of postoperative pain and severe pain (VAS >7) among third and fourth degree haemorrhoids.

Postoperative symptoms duration including pain, bleeding, soiling and hitching lasted more after CH compared to SH reaching significant differences for soiling and bleeding (please refer to figure 3).

Postoperative fever was similar between the two groups. No differences were observed in terms of return to work expressed in days between the SH and CH.

Urgency after 3 months was significantly more frequent after SH compared to CH (8.2% vs 0.6%), despite this difference disappeared at 1 year (0.9% vs 0.3%).

Three patients (2.7%) experienced severe disabling chronic pain after SH that lasted >1 year since surgery without the expected improvement over the follow-up. Early haemorrhoidal recurrences (as thrombosis) occurred 4 and 12 days after surgery. Six patients developed late haemorrhoidal recurrence after 16±5 months from previous surgery. Twelve patients experienced transient urgency (10.9%) that resolved within 4 months in all patients but one in which lasted 13 months. Two patients (1.8%) developed symptomatic rectal stricture with urgency and frequency and responded to anal dilatation with anal dilators. Overall reinterventions rate after SH was 9.1% (vs 4.8% of CH, not significant).

INTRODUCTION

Haemorrhoids are common, and approximately 10 to 20% of symptomatic patients require surgery [1]. Conventional haemorrhoidectomy (CH) by open or closed excision is still the most common and definitive treatment of prolapsed third- or fourth-degree haemorrhoids. Among those, Milligan-Morgan, Ferguson and Parks operations are widely applied surgical procedures in the colorectal practice, being theoretically simple, very effective and reasonable safe [2]. On the other hand, CH is followed by an unpleasant postoperative period often accompanied by considerable pain and delayed patient's recovery and return to normal activities. Excessive dissection and the use of diathermy or sutures on highly vascularized tissue are pointed as responsible for this.

Stapled haemorrhoidopexy (SH) is an attractive alternative to CH because of reduced postoperative pain, shorter hospital stay and earlier return to normal activities [3,4]. Over the last decade, SH gained wide acceptance as an effective, safe and less painful technique to treat haemorrhoids. It can be performed in a day-surgery setting, and some authors suggested that this could reduce the overall cost of the procedure [5]. Based on existing literature, over 50,000 patients have been treated in Europe, and this technique seems to be indicated for all haemorrhoid degrees [6].

However, this enthusiastic use has been tempered by increasing reports of unusual complications, including several cases of pelvic life threatening sepsis and deaths [5,6]. Although several complications are similar to CH, some are technique-related such as longer-term anal pain (post-evacuation syndrome or persistent anal pain), longer-term tenesmus with urgency and/or frequency, haemorrhoidal recurrence (early as thrombosis or late recurrences), recto-vaginal fistula, anastomotic leakage, rectal perforation and pelvic sepsis [7-9].

In this chapter we report data from a prospective study on stapled haemorroidopexy including the management of complications. We also correlate pathological findings to short- and long-term clinical outcomes. All results are compared to a cohort of patients who underwent conventional haemorrhoidectomy.

PATIENTS AND METHODS

Between January 2003 and October 2007, 425 symptomatic patients underwent haemorrhoidectomy at our Institution and data entered prospectively in a database. Of those, 110 underwent SH (66 M, 44 F, mean age 44 years, ranging from 21 to 75 years) while 315 underwent conventional haemorrhoidectomy (186 M, 129 F, mean age 48 ranging from 24 to 72 years).

All procedures were performed by two colorectal surgeons (PS and VMS). Cases performed as emergency procedures or performed by residents as part of the teaching program were excluded from this study. Patients with inflammatory bowel disease, coexisting anorectal disease, or previous anal surgery were excluded as well. Patients requiring concomitant anorectal or pelvic floor surgery in addition to haemorrhoidectomy were also excluded.

Mean follow-up period after surgery was similar between the two groups being respectively 25±14 months after SH and 32±16 months after CH. Before surgery, all patients underwent digital examination and proctoscopy. Preoperative Wexner continence score was performed in all patients. Colonoscopy, anorectal manometry and/or ultrasonography (US) were performed if necessary. All surgeries were performed in a Day Care setting, in lithotomic position under local anaesthesia and, when necessary, general anaesthesia was provided. All patients received a phosphate enema 2 h before the operation. Antibiotic prophylaxis was administered using intravenous cephalosporin (1 gr) and metronidazole (500 mg) immediately before surgery. Starting May 2006 our protocol was revised and a single-antibiotic regimen replaced the previous one using intravenous cefotaxime (2 gr).

The procedure was performed according to the technique described by Longo [8] using the PPH01 kit (Ethicon Endo-Surgery) with no modifications or additional procedures until 2008 when PPH02 kit (Ethicon Endo-Surgery) was introduced in use.

Mucosal doughnuts retrieved from the stapler were orientated and sent for pathology examination in 10% neutral buffered formalin. All specimens were reviewed by a single consultant pathologist. The macroscopic appearance of each resected specimen, including shape, size, and depth, was recorded.

Microscopically, the presence of columnar, transitional, and squamous epithelium, as well as involvement of circular and longitudinal smooth muscle, was assessed. Smooth muscle beneath the squamous epithelium was considered to represent internal anal sphincter. Features of mucosal prolapse, such as muscularization of the lamina propria, thickening/disruption of the muscularis mucosa, diamond-shaped crypts, surface hyperplasia, and thrombosed vessels, were also assessed [9].

Patients were discharged from the unit 4 to 8 h after the procedure with oral and written instructions for postoperative care including medications (nonsteroidal anti-inflammatory drugs per os), antibiotics (quinolones twice a day for 5 days per os) and stool softeners for 7 days. Warm sitz baths were suggested.

Patients were seen after 1 week and pain assessed using a 10-cm (centimeters) linear visual analogue scale (VAS). Further controls were scheduled at 1, 3 and 12 months or if required. All patients were contacted annually thereafter. Clinical outcome was assessed by a validated questionnaire on postoperative symptoms and satisfaction supplemented by the Wexner continence score.

Data on bleeding, body temperature, pain after defecation, prolapse, incontinence, and fecal urgency were recorded and prospectively entered in a database. Patients with delayed healing, chronic pain, or complicated outcome underwent anorectal manometry and/or US. Data were analysed using Fisher exact and Mann–Whitney tests. We evaluated the association between considered variables using odds ratio estimate with 95% confidence limits.

During the same period of time, 23 patients were referred to our colorectal unit after complicated CH or SH performed elsewhere: six after CH (four F, two M) and 17 (eleven F, six M; mean age 47 years) after SH. The onset and duration of specific SH-related complications as well as reinterventions for failed and or complicated SH were recorded.

RESULTS

One-hundred-six operations were carried out as planned day-case surgery, whereas four patients were admitted to the hospital (3.6%) at the end of the day. Indications for hospitalization were severe pain, urinary retention and the need for longer patient observation as recommended by the anaesthesiologist when surgery was performed later in the day. The median hospital stay for these patients was 1.3 days, ranging from 1 to 4 days. None required further surgical intervention.

Operating time between SH and CH was similar being 28.3±8.7 and 26±8.8 min, respectively ($p=0.111$). Hospitalization rates were similar between SH and CH being 2.7% and 1.6%, respectively ($p=0.449$).

Likewise, no differences were observed in terms of ER (Emergency Room) admissions (7.3% vs 3.8%, $p=0.214$) and hospital readmissions (3.6% and 2.2%, $p=0.414$) between SH and CH.

Early and Late Complications: Overall early (<30 days from surgery) and late (>30 days) complication rates were similar between SH and CH as shown in Tables 1 and 2.

Table 1. Early Complications (<30 days)

Complications	SH (n/%)	CH (n/%)	P value
Urinary retention	3/2.7%	5/1.6%	0.449
Bleeding	5/4.5%	9/2.8%	0.394
Faecal retention	1/0.9%	5/1.6%	0.604
Haem. thrombosis	2/1.8%	1/0.3%	0.106
Incontinence	3/2.7%	7/2.2%	0.090
Infection	0	3/0.9%	0.305
Overall	14/12.7%	30/9.5%	0.343

Table 2. Late Complications

Complications	SH (n/%)	CH (n/%)	P value
Disabling pain (>1 year)	3/2.7%	2/0.6%	0.082
Recurrence	6/5.4%	5/1.6%	0.133
Stenosis	2/1.8%	10/1.2%	0.460
Anal fissure	6/5.4%	7/2.2%	0.090
Abscess/fistula	0	2/0.6%	0.403
Skin tags	13/11.8%	41/13.2%	0.746
Overall	30/27.2%	67/21.2%	0.197

Three SH patients visited the Emergency Department overnight because of urinary retention. All of them required urinary catheterization and one was readmitted after 2 days and required the placement of a Foley catheter that was removed 3 days later in an outpatient clinic.

Five patients in SH group visited the Emergency Department from 2 to 20 days (2, 5, 5, 7 and 20 days) after surgery because of bleeding. These patients had undergone surgery for third- (two) and fourth- (three) degree hemorrhoids, and in all cases, pathology revealed a full thickness resection. Three were admitted, and a Foley catheter was inserted into the anorectal canal to compress the bleeding vessels. This procedure was effective in all cases but one, which required surgical revision. None of the patients required blood transfusions.

Overall median hospital stay for readmitted patients was 3 days, ranging from 2 to 5 days. Postoperative fever was similar between the two groups. No differences were observed in terms of return to work expressed in days between the two groups.

Longer-term follow-up results of symptoms duration is shown in Table 3.

Despite an increased quote of anal fissure, disabling chronic pain and recurrences were observed after SH when compared to CH, no significative differences were observed in terms of early and late complications between SH and CH as shown in Tables 1 and 2.

Mean pain during the first postoperative week expressed as VAS is shown in Figure 1. Significant differences were observed from postoperative days 4 to 7.

As shown in Figure 2, patients who underwent CH experienced more severe pain (expressed as VAS score>7) than SH at 5, 6 and 7 postoperative days. We did not observed differences between SH and CH in terms of postoperative pain and severe pain (VAS>7) among third and fourth degree haemorrhoids.

Postoperative symptoms duration including pain, bleeding, soiling and hitching lasted more after CH compared to SH reaching significant differences for soiling and bleeding as shown in Figure 3.

Table 3. Longer-term follow-up and symptoms duration

Parameter	SH (n/%)	CH (n/%)	P value
Fever (> 38°C)	4/3.6%	14/4.4%	0.821
Bleeding at 3/12	2/1.8%	5/1.6%	0.870
Urgency at 3/12	9/8.2%	2/0.6%	0.045
Pain at 3/12	3/2.7%	4/1.2%	0.175
Bleeding at 1 yr	1/0.9%	2/0.6%	0.967
Urgency at 1 yr	1/0.9%	1/0.3%	0.436
Pain at 1 yr	3/2.7%	2/0.6%	0.082
Satisfaction (score 4/4)	85%	66%	0.051
Return to work (days)	17.3±11.7	17.5±10.8	0.856

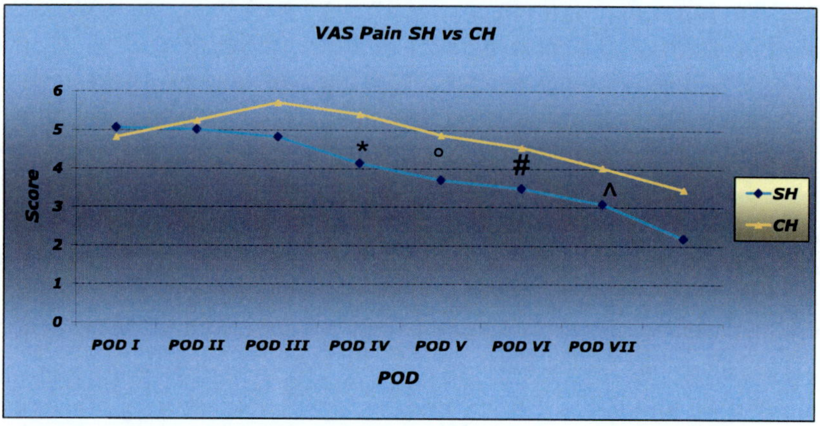

* p = 0.0004; ° p = 0.003; # p = 0.003; ^ p = 0.001

Figure 1. Pain SH (expressed as VAS score mean)

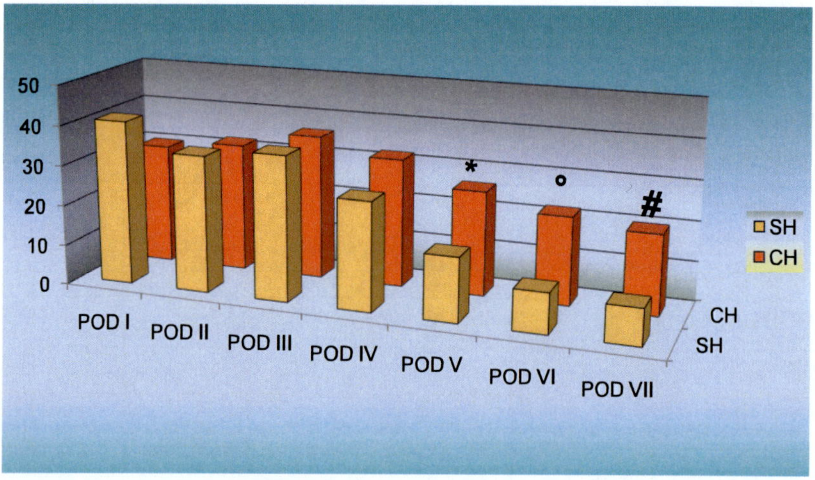

* p = 0.02; ° p = 0.005; # p = 0.008

Figure 2. Severe postoperative pain (expressed as % of patients with VAS>7)

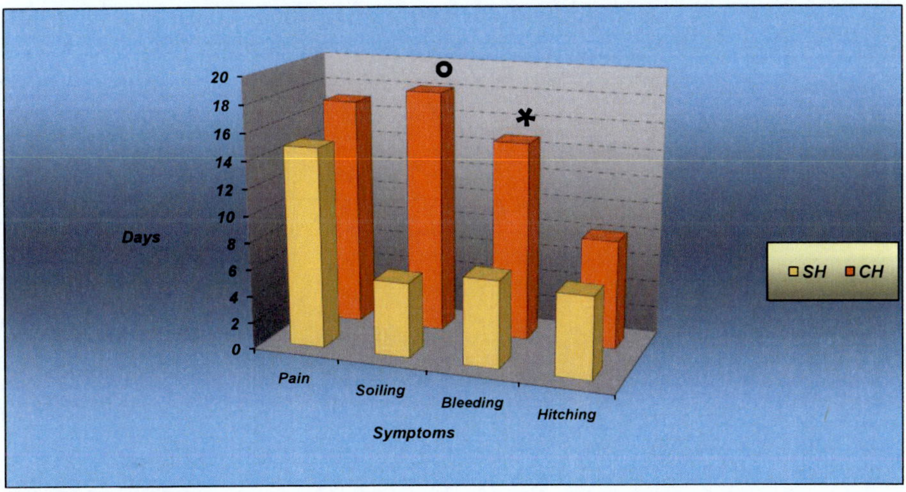

° p=0.042; * p=0.002

Figure 3. Postoperative Symptoms Duration

Urgency after 3 months was significantly more frequent after SH compared to CH (8.2% vs 0.6%), despite this difference disappeared at 1 year (0.9% vs 0.3%).

Three patients (2.7%) experienced severe disabling chronic pain after SH that lasted >1 year since surgery without the expected improvement over the follow-up. All patients described the pain as sharp, recurrent, starting within 30 min from defecation and lasting for 2 to 5 h without bleeding or mucous discharge. In all cases, the rectal examination was unremarkable and anal fissure was ruled out. All patients underwent anal manometry that did not show significant abnormalities (only one patient was found to have mild internal anal sphincter hypertonia) as well as endorectal ultrasound that showed normal anatomy in all. A working diagnosis of post-defecation syndrome was made in all and calcium channel blockers ointment given twice a day for 8 weeks. This treatment was effective in all but one who presented worsening persistent pain described as sharper after defecation. In this case oral nifedipine was ineffective and anorectal exploration under anaesthesia was performed. At surgery, the staple line was correctly placed and the only finding was the presence of retained staples which were removed with complete pain resolution within 2 weeks.

SH complications and their management resumé is shown in Table 4.

Early haemorrhoidal recurrences (as thrombosis) occurred 4 and 12 days after surgery.

Table 4. SH complications and management resume

Complications	Number (n)	Management	n/%
Bleeding	5	Conservative Surgery	4/5 1
Thrombosis (at POD 4 and 12)	2	Conservative	Effective
Disabling pain (US, MRI, Manometry)	3	Analgesic/Ca2+ CB EUA	Topical (1) Oral (1) Stapler removal effective (1)
Recurrence (16±5 months)	6	Medical/RBL Surgery-CH	1/2 RBL effective 1 refused 2 Closed/2 Open
Fissure	6	Medical (GTN) Surgery	Effective 4/6 (66.7%) 2 LIS, effective
Stenosis	2	Dilators	Effective

Both cases responded to standard medical treatment and did not present any other episode during the follow-up. Six patients developed late haemorrhoidal recurrence after 16±5 months from previous surgery (range 9–26 months). All recurrences were observed in patients who underwent SH for fourth degree haemorrhoids. Main symptoms were bleeding (six patients) and prolapse (four patients). One patient was successfully treated with rubber banding while surgery was offered to the remaining five: one patient refused and four underwent uneventful CH (two closed and two open).

Twelve patients experienced transient urgency (10.9%) that resolved within 4 months in all patients but one in which lasted 13 months. Two patients (1.8%) developed symptomatic rectal stricture with urgency and frequency and responded to anal dilatation with anal dilators. As shown in Table 5, overall reinterventions rate after SH was 9.1% (vs 4.8% of CH, not significant).

Figure 4 shows the estimated risk of reinterventions after SH and CH.

Pathology: Macroscopic appearance of specimens was rectangular with a median size of 3.98+/−1.54 by 2.1+/−0.8 cm. Median depth was 1.11+/−0.34 cm, ranging from 0.1 to 2 cm.

Table 5. Number of patients with a complication (N) requiring reintervention (n)

Reintervention	SH n/N (%)	CH n/N (%)	P value
For pain	1/3(33.3%)	0/2	0.83
For bleeding	1/5(20%)	3/9(33.33%)	0.54
For skin tags	2/13(15.4%)	3/41(7.3%)	0.39
For anal fissure	2/6(33%)	4/7(57%)	0.43
For abscess/Fistula	0	2/2(100%)	0.79
For stenosis	0/2	2/10(20%)	0.84
For recurrence	4/8(50%)	1/5(20%)	0.31
Cumulative	10/37(27%)	15/74(20.3%)	0.64
OVERALL RATE	10/110(9.1%)	15/315(4.8%)	0.06

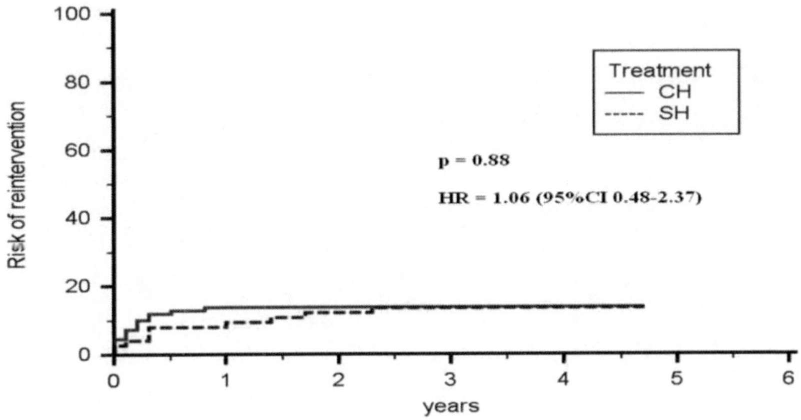

Figure 4. Estimated risk of reinterventions after SH and CH

Pathology revealed that 100% of the specimens contained columnar mucosa: 54.6% contained only columnar epithelium; 32.7% contained columnar and transitional epithelium; and 12.7% contained columnar, anal transitional, and stratified squamous epithelium (Figure 5). Smooth muscle was observed in 57.3% of the specimens (Figure 6).

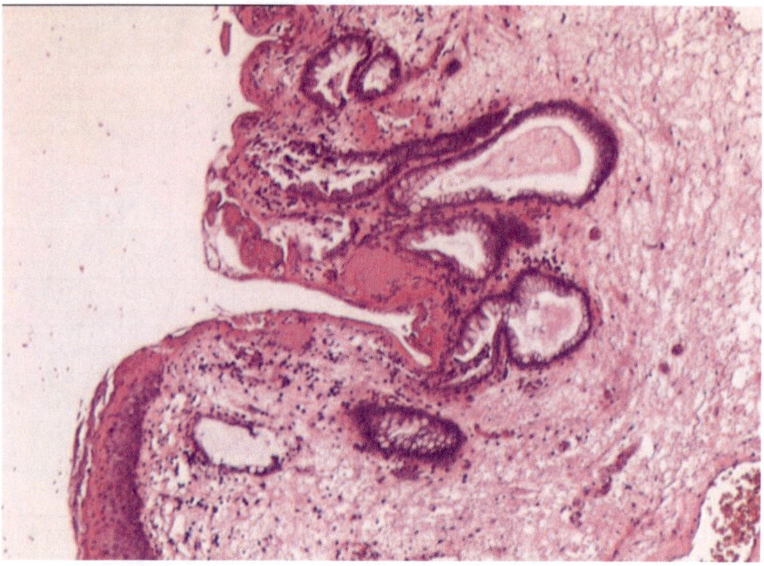

Figure 5. Resected specimen histology: transitional epithelium, diamond shape crypts, ulcers

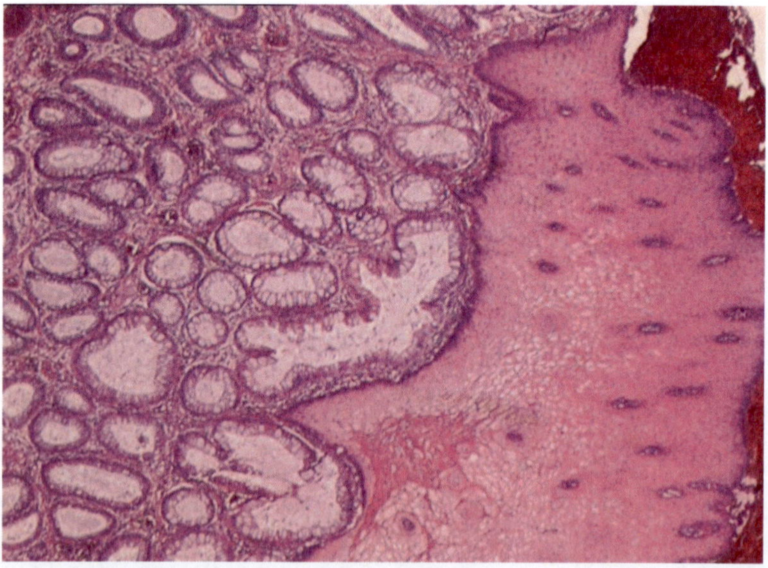

Figure 6. Resected specimen histology: transitional and squamous epithelium above smooth circular muscle (internal sphincter)

Table 6. Histology of the resected specimens divided by genders and statistical significance

Pathology findings		Male	Female	P value
Epithelium n/(%)				
columnar only	60 (54.6%)	36 (60%)	24 (40%)	NS
+ transitional	36 (32.7%)	21 (58.3%)	15 (41.7%)	NS
+ transitional, and squamous	14 (12.7%)	9 (64.2%)	5 (33.3%)	0.05
Smooth muscle				
circular only	51 (46.4%)	28 (54.9%)	23 (45.8%)	NS
+ longitudinal	12 (10.9%)	8 (66.7%)	4 (33.3%)	0.05
total	63 (57.3%)	36 (57.2%)	27 (42.8%)	NS

Table 7. Correlation Between Pathology Findings and Postoperative Pain (n=Number of Patients with Specific Pathology Finding and Pain; N=Total Number of Patients with Specific Pathology Finding) [38].

Pathology findings/pain	1 week *n/N*	1 month *n/N*	3 months *n/N*	1 year *n/N*
Epithelium				
Columnar only	3/54 (NA)	6/54 (NA)	2/54 (NA)	1/54 (NA)
+ Transitional	0/28 (NA)	12/28 (OR=4.5; CL=1.55 & 12.93)	7/28 (OR_1=9; CL=1.7 & 47)	2/28 (NA)
+ Transitional, and squamous	1/12 (NA)	0/12 (NA)	2/12 (OR_2=6, NS)	0 (NA)
Smooth muscle				
Yes	0/59 (NA)	9/59 (OR=0.4, NS)	7/59 (OR=1.0, NS)	2/59 (NA)

Circular smooth muscle was present in 46.4%, whereas longitudinal smooth muscle was present in 10.9%. All samples contained at least one feature of prolapse. Table 6 shows the distribution of squamous epithelium and smooth muscle between genders. Our findings showed significant differences between males and females regarding the presence of squamous epithelium and longitudinal smooth muscle in the resected specimen.

A significant association between longer-term pain and the presence of transitional epithelium in the specimen was observed (Table 7). Although a trend in increased postoperative pain if squamous epithelium was also present was observed, this was not significant. No correlation or differences were observed if smooth muscle was present. Squamous epithelium and smooth muscle were both present (indicating the presence of internal sphincter fibers) in six patients (five males and one female). Of those, two experienced longer-term pain and one experienced incontinence. The presence of squamous and/or transitional epithelium and circular or longitudinal smooth muscle in the specimen was not associated with the clinical findings of fecal urgency, tenesmus, or soiling.

Referred patients: Among the referred SH group, one patient developed severe pelvic sepsis after SH performed as a day case procedure. She complained lower quadrants abdominal pain associated to nausea, vomit and fever the night following hospital discharge. She was admitted in our emergency unit because of acute abdomen. Signs of severe sepsis were present and computed tomography (CT) scan showed pneumoretroperitoneum. At laparotomy, mesorectal and retroperitoneal emphysema were present with minimal amount of pus, in absence of an evident low rectal perforation. After accurate washout, a Hartman's procedure was performed and a drain left in the pelvis. Postoperative recovery was uneventful, she was discharged after 8 days and uneventful reversal was performed 6 months later.

Ten of the remaining 16 patients experienced at least one of the following symptoms or complications: recurrence (6), urgency (6), severe chronic anal pain (4), tenesmus (4), colicky abdominal pain (1), anal fissure (1) and stenosis (1).

Recurrences were observed after 17±6 months from surgery (range 9 to 36 months). Main symptoms were bleeding (six patients), prolapse (four patients) and pain (one patient). Four patients accepted surgery and underwent conventional haemorrhoidectomy (three closed, one open) and had a regular postoperative recovery.

Four patients came to our attention because of persistent pain lasting for 7±6 months after SH. In one case, an anal fissure was present and successfully treated with lateral internal sphincterotomy after manometric confirmation of internal sphincter hypertonia and failure of GTN ointment course of 8 weeks. Topical treatment with calcium channel blockers ointment (twice a day for 8 weeks) was started in all. One patient required oral nifedipine. However, conservative medical treatment was ineffective in two patients, who underwent exploration under anaesthesia (EUA). Before reinterventions anorectal manometry and ultrasound were performed in both and pelvic magnetic resonance imaging (MRI) in one. In one patient, the US showed a small (1 cm) submucosal abscess at the stapled line. The abscess was not seen at the MRI, and it was not found at EUA. However, in both patients, surgical removal of retained staples resolved the pain within 4 weeks. One referred patient with anorectal stricture underwent anoplasty. In this case, asymmetric, very low stapled line was observed at surgery. Table 8 shows summary of complications and management among the referred patients.

Patients' satisfaction at longer-term follow-up was 85% in SH group and 66% after CH (p=0.051).

Table 8. (Referred patients): Summary of complications and management

Complications	Number (n)	Management	Notes/Outcome
Rectal perforation	1	Hartmann	Reversed 4/12 later
Tenesmus-Urgency	10	Biofeedback	
Disabling chronic pain	4	Analgesic/Ca^{2+} CB EUA (stapler removal)	Uneffective 2/4 Effective 2/2
Recurrence	6	Conservative RB Surgery-CH	Uneffective 6/6 Effective 1/2 4 (3 closed/1 open)
Stenosis	1	Anoplasty	Asymmetric low stapled line
Fissure	1	Medical (GTN) Surgery (LIS)	Uneffective Effective

DISCUSSION

Stapled haemorrhoidopexy allows removal of a circular section of prolapsed rectal mucosa with immediate mucoso–mucosal anastomosis, achieving a lifting effect for haemorrhoidal cushions and restoring their physiological position [8]. The interruption of the arteriovenous communications may also reduce engorgement of the haemorrhoidal vascular cushions. Moreover, the succeeding deep fibrosis of the stapled line may play a role in maintaining the reduction [10]. Because the suture line is located between 3 and 5 cm from the dentate line, sensory nerve endings are not compromised with significant reduction of postoperative pain when compared to conventional haemorrhoidectomy (either open or closed). Thus, by resecting the rectal mucosa only, the anal canal sensation is unaffected.

Several reports have shown that this innovative approach is safe, effective, and advantageous in terms of reduced pain and faster return to normal activities. As a consequence, over the last decade, we have contributed to an impressive widespread use of this technique.

Recently, this enthusiasm has been tempered by longer-term results and increasing reports of severe septic complications and deaths.

Complications rates of SH range from 6.4% to 31% [11,12] with a reintervention rate after 1 year of 11% [13]. Some complications are similar to conventional haemorrhoidectomy such as bleeding, urinary retention, incontinence, fissure and stenosis. Others are specific-related to the technique, such as intra-abdominal or retroperitoneal bleeding, pelvic sepsis, tenesmus, severe chronic anal pain (chronic proctalgia or postdefecation syndrome), rectovaginal fistula and damage to sphincterial mechanism [14–17].

Accurate placement of the staple line is mandatory to avoid internal anal sphincter and anodermal tissue involvement [18]. Ideally, as indicated by Shanmugam et al., the resected doughnut should only contain columnar epithelium [19]. If the purse-string suture is performed too low, close to the dentate line, the specimen will contain transitional and/or squamous epithelium with possible increase in postoperative pain. Nevertheless, if the purse string includes the smooth muscle layer that encircles the anal canal, damage to the sphincterial apparatus may occur with continence impairment. On the other hand, if the stapled line is placed too high, the procedure will be ineffective.

Efficacy and Safety: Our experience confirms that SH is followed by reduced postoperative pain during the first week, with overall early and late complications rates similar to CH.

Pain: Postoperative pain (scored according to VAS) was significantly lower after SH compared to CH starting from POD 4. Our results confirm that SH procedure causes significantly less postoperative pain than CH, mostly during the first week and beyond up to four weeks after surgery [1]. This leads to a lesser requirement for analgesics after SH compared to CH both during the hospital stay and after the discharge [20].

Wound discharge and recovery: Postoperative symptoms duration is shorter after SH with a better patients satisfaction compared to CH. This faster surgical (in terms of local symptoms) and functional (in terms of recovery and return to work) is common and well established from several systematic reviews. Wound healing occurs within 4 weeks and return to work is commonly faster (1 weeks earlier compared to CH). Similarly return to normal activities is about 2 weeks earlier compared to CH [1]. However, differently from these results, in our experience the mean return to work period (expressed in days) was similar between SH and CH [11–13]. We explain this similarity of results with the fact the our hospital serves a large Government employed (directly or indirectly) population with paid sick leave. As a consequence, in addition to surgical expertise, Institutional and Government guidelines as well as social culture could account for variation in the length of hospital stay or time to return to works observed in several reports [1].

Bleeding: The most common complication after SH is postoperative bleeding, which is reported between 2 and 28% [4,12,17]. We observed a 4.5% rate of bleeding requiring admission. A second operation was needed in 20% of cases. According to existing literature, bleeding is rarely life-threatening and can be successfully managed by the insertion of a Foley catheter in the anorectal canal, local adrenaline injection or enema. The need of reintervention is rare [12] but this risk seems to be higher after SH [20]. Our bleeding incidence is low if compared to the incidence reported in existing literature. Careful inspection of the staple line at the end of the operation should be mandatory, and any bleeding vessel should be coagulated with diathermy or oversewn with absorbable stitches. Bleeding events in our series occurred late after surgery, up to 20 days after. Although several authors have shown an increased risk of postoperative bleeding after SH for fourth-degree hemorrhoids, in our experience the incidence of bleeding in third- and fourth-degree hemorrhoids did not differ significantly [6,21]. On the other hand, the incidence of bleeding was significantly higher if a full-thickness resection was accidentally performed, as demonstrated by pathology.

Blouhos et al. reported a case of uncontrollable intraabdominal bleeding necessitating low anterior rectal resection because of a small laceration in the anterior aspect of the rectum [22]

Sepsis: The most dangerous complication reported after SH is pelvic sepsis, usually subsequent to rectal perforation or anastomotic leak. In a recent systematic review of life-threatening sepsis following haemorrhoidectomy, McCloud et al. described seven cases of life-threatening complications between 2000 and 2003 including abscesses, fistulae, retroperitoneal sepsis and rectal perforations as well as pneumoretroperitoneum and pneumomediastinum [7]. Six patients required faecal diversion, and one died. These reports tempered the initial enthusiasm for SH and in 2004 Nisar et al. emphasized "potentially devastating complications" of SH in a meta-analysis indicating CH as the gold standard [23]. Since then, an equal number of life-threatening complications after SH have also been reported, the majority requiring faecal diversion with occasional deaths. The number of these adverse events is comparable to those observed after CH over a 40 year period (1964–2003), although severe complications following CH hardly require faecal diversion [24]. Pescatori et al. observed that the risk of these severe complications is higher after SH because it involves the distal rectum with a 'blind' resection and suture, close to the vagina, the prostate and the Douglas pouch, which is also a possible site of an enterosigmoidocele [24]. Although Ravo et al. estimated a life-threatening complications rate of 1:1200 after SH in a large retrospective study, we believe that the real number of life-threatening complications is largely overlooked because of unpublished events. It has been pointed that most of these cases have been performed by general surgeons [24] despite the fact that a consensus paper had recommended that the operation should be carried out only by specialists trained in this technique [25]. In case of unexpected severe perineal or abdominal pain, urinary retention or difficulties with micturition, fever and leucocytosis, even if local examination is negative, an abdominal CT scan should be immediately performed. Predominant findings at CT scan are pneumoretroperitoneum, pneumomediastinum and subcutaneous emphysema [26,27]. Despite the fact that successful conservative management has been reported, we believe that anastomotic repair with faecal diversion or a Hartman's procedure should always be performed before worsening of clinical conditions. At exploration (by laparotomy or laparoscopy), very little will be found with oedema of the rectum and pararectal tissues associated to minimal or absent retroperitoneal fluid or pus, depending from the onset and duration of symptoms prior surgery. Emphysema along the mesorectum and retroperitoneum can be observed.

We did not observe any secondary infection of the stapled line, likely because of the longer antibiotic prophylaxis (extended for 5 days after surgery) compared to other case series in which infection of the staple line has been reported.

Recto-vaginal fistula can also occur, and to date three cases have been described [14,28,29]. This complication can be avoided by assessing the thickness of the rectovaginal septum before inserting the purse-string suture. Care should be taken not to place too deep a suture anteriorly during the purse-string, and vagina should be examined before firing. If rectovaginal fistula occurs, immediate repair should be attempted after excision of the staples ring, and a faecal diversion should be made.

Obstruction: Three cases of acute rectal obstruction after SH have been reported worldwide secondary to complete closure of the distal rectum by the retained purse string entrapped by the staples (two cases) or secondary to haematoma within the layers of the bowel wall (one case) [30–32]. It may require laparotomy and faecal diversion due to subsequent spontaneous or iatrogenic perforation. If immediately recognised a *Delorme* approach could be attempted [30].

Although we did not observe any, the rectal pocket syndrome may follow SH due to the entrapment of faecoliths leading to transient intramural sepsis [33]. This syndrome may be due to incorrect placement of purse-string suture and requires laying open the pocket [33].

Impairment of Sphincterial apparatus (incontinence, chronic pain, urgency): Several authors suggested possible lesions of the anal sphincterial apparatus mainly secondary to anal dilatation or muscle entrapment at stapler firing. Randomised data have shown that the continence score as well as anorectal manometric and endoanal US findings are similar to those found after CH [16].

The incidence of incontinence to gas, liquid or solid is extremely low after SH and similar to CH. Severe persistent pain after SH has been reported between 2% and 16%, and represents the most common cause of reintervention (up to 45% of cases) [13,21,24]. In absence of thrombosis or fissure, the pain is described as intense and dull, refractory to treatment and associated variably with tenesmus or urgency (proctalgia). However, pain can be sharp and rapidly increasing after defecation (10–30 min) without evidence of an anal fissure (post-defecation syndrome). Its aetiology is uncertain, and there is clinical evidence of anal sphincter spasm and high anal sphincter pressures on manometry [34]. Calcium channel blockers therapy is effective with restoration of quality of life [34]. In this report, a total of seven patients experienced persistent pain and all initially treated with topical and oral Calcium channel blockers. This treatment was effective in four who presented a clear post-defecation syndrome. Three patients required anal exploration under anaesthesia and, along with other authors, the surgical removal of the retained staples or stitches allowed complete resolution of the pain and associated symptoms [24]

Despite the fact that only columnar epithelium and no smooth muscle should be present in the specimen, in our series squamous epithelium was present in 12.7% of cases and full-thickness rectal wall in 11.9% of cases. George et al. observed the presence of internal anal sphincter muscle fibers in 38% of the doughnuts and full thickness rectal wall in 42% [9]. In a pathology audit of 106 SHs, Shanmugam et al. reported the inclusion of squamous epithelium in 18% of the cases and smooth muscle in 74.5%, while an involvement of the internal sphincter occurred in 5.6% of the cases [19]. If the smooth muscle layer beneath the squamous epithelium is considered to be part of the internal anal sphincter, in our series it was retrieved in six cases, mostly in male patients (five out of six).

Correlation between pathology and postoperative pain showed that it was increased if squamous and transitional epithelium were present in the specimen. The presence of smooth muscle seems to be irrelevant with respect to postoperative pain, but if squamous epithelium and smooth muscle are both present (indicating the presence of internal sphincter fibers), longer-term pain (two patients) and incontinence (one patient) can be observed. Even other authors have indicated that inclusion of smooth muscle in the excised doughnut may be related to the subsequent development of pain, despite clear data are not available [12]. Mlakar et al. suggested that severe longer-term pain may be related to haemostatic stitches at the staple line close to the dentate line [12]. It can be speculated that the metallic staples may act as ongoing inflammatory stimulus responsible for longer term pain [35]. Accurate placement of the staple line is mandatory in order to avoid internal anal sphincter and anodermal tissue involvement [17].

Tenesmus, frequency and faecal urgency are variably associated and reported between 5% and 40% and are usually transient and self-limiting [11–14]. These symptoms were observed in about 14.5% of our patients, but both tenesmus and urgency were the most frequent complications in the referred group.

According to other authors, we believe that they may arise because of tissue oedema and thrombosis as well as disruption of the anatomy and function of the normal anal cushions as follow-up examination usually do not demonstrate any abnormality such as low placement of the staple line or damage to the dentate line and are usually transitory.

However, the reduced rectal capacity may explain frequency and urgency increase as well as tenesmus as observed by Pescatori and Chetham [15,24].

The presence of transitional or squamous epithelium or the presence of circular or longitudinal smooth muscle in the specimen does not correlate to the clinical findings of fecal urgency, tenesmus, or postoperative soiling.

Urinary retention: Our incidence of urinary retention was 2.7%, similar to that reported in literature (1.5 to 8%) [17,21]. Theoretically, the lower postoperative pain should make urethral sphincter spasm unlikely, but, in fact, the incidence of urinary retention is as high as it is in conventional hemorrhoidectomy. Despite a trend favouring SH in the development of postoperative urinary retention exists, this difference is not significant as shown in several meta-analysis [1]. The causes of postoperative urinary retention are unclear.

Early and Late recurrences: According to existing literature, recurrent prolapse as well as the need of reintervention are more common after SH than CH, especially if SH is performed to treat fourth degree haemorrhoids [36].

We observed a high rate of residual and recurrent haemorrhoids (6.3%). Shalaby and Desoky reported a 1% recurrent prolapse, but this study included also patients with second degree haemorrhoids [4,11,16,26]. Conversely, Ganio et al. reported a 20% recurrent prolapse after a telephone follow-up on 50 patients who underwent SH [4]. All our recurrences occurred in patients with fourth-degree haemorrhoids. Similarly, Ortiz et al. reported more frequent recurrence in fourth-degree haemorrhoids compared to third-degree [37]. In our experience, recurrence rate after CH is less than 2% (five out 315 patients) for similar follow-up of SH without differences between third-degree (three patients out of 196) and fourth-degree (two patients out of 119) haemorrhoids. These findings persuaded us to believe that fourth degree haemorrhoids may not represent an appropriate indication for SH, as the success of the operation depends entirely on the resection and reduction of the prolapse by the staple. Since May 2006, we have reserved SH to third-degree haemorrhoids only and, despite a shorter follow-up compared to the entire group, we did not observe any recurrence to date.

Conclusions

Our experience confirms that this technique is feasible and safe when performed as a day-surgery procedure for third-degree hemorrhoids. However, the risk of severe life-threatening complications and frequent recurrences explain the reduced use of this technique to treat haemorrhoidal disease. Because of this potential for specific technique-related complications, it should not be used for second-degree hemorrhoids, whereas for fourth-degree hemorrhoids conventional excision might be more effective, reducing the incidence of longer-term recurrence. Nevertheless longer-term and larger studies are needed to further clarify its indications; meanwhile, abuses should be minimised to reduce unusual and challenging complications.

The correct placement of the purse-string suture is mandatory to avoid postoperative pain, and pathological examination of the resected specimen should always be performed. Only columnar epithelium should be present in the specimen and, although the presence of smooth muscle does not influence the outcome in terms of functional results, it may play a role in postoperative bleeding.

References

[1] Tjandra J, Chan KY. Systematic Review on the Procedure for Prolapse and Hemorrhoids (Stapled Hemorrhoidopexy). *Dis. Colon. Rectum.* 2007;50:878–892.

[2] Leventoglu S, Mentes B, Akin M and Oguz M. Haemorrhoidectomy with electrocautery or ultrashears and stapled haemorrhoidopexy. *ANZ J. Surg.* 2008;78:389–393.

[3] Roswell M, Bello M, Hemingway DM. Circumferential mucosectomy versus conventional haemorrhoidectomy: randomised controlled trial. *Lancet* 2000;355:779–781.

[4] Ganio E, Altomare DF, Gabrielli F, Milito G, Canuti S. Prospective randomized multicentre trial comparing stapled and open haemorrhoidectomy. *Br. J. Surg.*2002;88:669–674.

[5] Slawik S, Kenefick N, Greenslade L, Dixon AR. A prospective evaluation of stapled haemorrhoidopexy/rectal mucosectomy in the management of 3rd and 4th degree haemorrhoids. *Colorectal Dis.* 2006;9:352–356.

[6] Finco C, Sarzo G, Savastano S, Degregori S, Merigliano S. Stapled haemorrhoidopexy in fourth degree haemorrhoidal prolapse: is it worthwhile? *Colorectal Dis* 2005;8:130–134.

[7] McCloud JM, Jameson JS, Scott ND. Life-threating sepsis following treatment for haemorrhoids: a systematic review. *Colorectal Dis.* 2006;8:748–755.

[8] Longo A. Treatment of haemorrhoids disease by reduction of mucosa and haemorrhoidal prolapse with a circular suturing device: a new procedure. In: *Proceedings of the 6th World Congress of Endoscopic Surgery*, Rome, 1998, pp 777–784.

[9] George BD, Shetty D, Lindsey I, Mortensen NJ, Warren BF. Histopathology of stapled haemorrhoidectomy specimens: a cautionary note. *Colorectal Dis* 2001;4:473–476.

[10] Beattie GC, McAdam TK, McIntosh SA, Loudon MA. Day case stapled haemorrhoidopexy for prolapsing haemorrhoids. *Colorectal Dis.* 2005;8:56–61.

[11] Kanellos I, Zacharakis E, Kanellos D, Pramateftakis MG, Tsachalis T, Betsis D. Long-term results after stapled haemorrhoidopexy for third-degree haemorrhoids. *Tech. Coloproctol.* 2006;10:47–49.

[12] Mlakar B, Kosorok P. Complications and results after stapled haemorrhoidopexy as a day surgical procedure. *Tech. Coloproctol.* 2003;7:164–168.

[13] Brusciano L, Ayabaca SM, Pescatori M et al. Reinterventions after complicated or failed stapled haemorrhoidopexy. *Dis. Colon. Rectum.* 2004;47:1846–1851.

[14] McDonald PJ, Bona R, Cohen CRG. Rectovaginal fistula after stapled haemorrhoidopexy. *Colorectal Dis.* 2004;6:64–65. letter.

[15] Cheetham MJ, Mortensen NJ, Nystrom PO, Kamm MA, Philips RKS. Persistent pain and fecal urgency after stapled haemorroidectomy. *Lancet* 2000;26:730–733.

[16] Ho YH, Seow-Cohen F, Tsang C, Eu KW. Randomized trial assessing anal sphincter injuries after stapled haemorrhoidectomy. *Br. J. Surg.* 2001;88:1449–1455.

[17] Oughriss M, Yver R, Faucheron JL. Complications of stapled haemorrhoidectomy: a french multicentric study. *Gastroenterol. Clin. Biol.* 2005;29:429–433.

[18] Corman ML, Graviè JF, Hager T, Loudon MA, Mascagni D, et al. Stapled haemorrhoidopexy: a consensus position paper by an international working party-indications, contra-indications and technique. *Colorectal. Dis.* 2003;5:304–310.

[19] Shanmugam V, Watson AJM, Chapman AD, Binnie NR, Loudon A. Pathological audit of stapled haemorrhoidopexy. *Colorectal Dis.* 2004;7:172–175.

[20] Shao WJ, Li G-CH, Zhang ZH-K, Yang B-L, Sun G-D and Chen Y-Q. Systematic review and meta-analysis of randomized controlled trials comparing stapled haemorrhoidopexy with conventional haemorrhoidectomy. *Br. J. Surg.* 2008; 95: 147–160.

[21] Ravo B, Amato A, Bianco V et al. Complications after stapled haemorrhoidectomy: can they be prevented? *Tech. Coloproctol.* 2003;6:83–88.

[22] Blouhos K, Vasiliadis K, Tsalis K, Botsios D, Vrakas X. Uncontrollable intra abdominal bleeding necessitating low anterior resection of the rectum after stapled haemorrhoidopexy: Report of a case. *Surg. Today* 2007;37(3):254–257.

[23] Nisar PJ, Acheson AG, Neal KR, Scholefield JH. Stapled haemorrhoidopexy compared with conventional haemorrhoidectomy: Systematic review of randomized, controlled trials. *Dis. Colon. Rectum.* 2004;47(11):1837–1845.

[24] Pescatori M, Aigner F. Stapled transanal rectal mucosectomy ten years after. *Tech. Coloproctol.* 2007;11(1):1–6.

[25] Corman ML, Gravié JF, Hager T, Loudon MA, Mascagni D, Nyström PO, Seow-Choen F, Abcarian H, Marcello P, Weiss E, Longo A. Stapled haemorrhoidopexy: A consensus position paper by an international working party—indications, contra-indications and technique. *Colorectal. Dis.* 2003;5(4):304–310.

[26] Ripetti V, Caricato M, Arullani A. Rectal perforation, retropneumoperitoneum, and pneumomediastinum after stapling procedure for prolapsed haemorrhoids: Report of a case and subsequent considerations. *Dis. Colon. Rectum* 2002;45(2):268–270.

[27] Filingeri V, Gravante G. Pneumoretroperitoneum, pneumomediastinum and subcutaneous emphysema of the neck after stapled haemorrhoidopexy. *Tech. Coloproctol.* 2005;9(1):86.

[28] Roos P. Haemorrhoid surgery revised. *Lancet* 2000;355 (9215):1648. May 6.

[29] Angelone G, Giardiello C, Prota C. Stapled haemorrhoidopexy. Complications and 2-year follow-up. *Chir. Ital.* 2006;58(6):753–760.

[30] Brown S, Baraza W, Shorthouse A. Total rectal lumen obliteration after stapled haemorrhoidopexy: a cautionary tale. *Tech. Coloproctol.* 2007; Nov 30.

[31] Cipriani S, Pescatori M. Acute rectal obstruction after PPH stapled haemorrhoidectomy. *Colorectal Dis.* 2002;4(5):367–370.

[32] Vasudevan SP, Mustafa el A, Gadhvi VM, Jhaldiyal P, Saharay M. Acute intestinal obstruction following stapled haemorrhoidopexy. *Colorectal. Dis.* 2007;9(7):668–669.

[33] Pescatori M, Spyrou M, Cobellis L, Bottini C, Tessera G. The rectal pocket syndrome after stapled mucosectomy. *Colorectal Dis.* 2006;8(9):808–811.

[34] Thaha MA, Irvine LA, Steele RJ, Campbell KL. Postdefaecation pain syndrome after circular stapled anopexy is abolished by oral nifedipine. *Br. J. Surg.* 2005;92(2):208–210.

[35] Filingeri V, Gravante G. Stapled haemorrhoidopexy followed by fecal urgency and tenesmus: methodological complication or surgeon's mistake? Correspondence *Tech. Coloproctol.* 2006;10:149–153.

[36] Ortiz H, Marzo J, Armendariz P, De Miguel M. Stapled hemorrhoidopexy *vs.* diathermy excision for fourth-degree hemorrhoids: a randomized, clinical trial and review of the literature. *Dis. Colon. Rectum* 2005;48:809–815.

[37] Ortiz H, Marzo J, Armendariz P. Randomised clinical trial of stapled haemorrhoidopexy versus conventional diathermy haemorrhoidectomy. *Br. J. Surg*. 2002;89:1376–1381.

[38] Stapled haemorrhoidopexy: a prospective study from pathology to clinical outcome.

Sileri P, Stolfi VM, Palmieri G, Mele A, Falchetti A, Di Carlo S, Gaspari AL *J Gastrointest Surg.* 2007 Dec; 11(12): 1662-8

In: Hemorrhoids: Symptoms, Diagnosis... ISBN: 978-1-60876-478-5
Authors: P. Salinitri et al., pp. 79-106

Chapter 4

HEMORRHOIDOPEXY USING PPH (PROCEDURE FOR PROLAPSE AND HEMORRHOIDS)

***Manousos-Georgios Pramateftakis*[1], *Dimitrios Kanellos*[2] *and Ioannis Kanellos*[1]**

[1] 4th Surgical Department, Aristotle University of Thessaloniki, Greece
[2] Surgical Department, Vivantes-Spandau Klinikum, Berlin, Germany

ABSTRACT

Hemorrhoidopathy is a common disease in the western world. It is believed that 20-30% of all people will develop symptomatic hemorrhoids at a stage of their life. It is one of the commonest benign pathologies that surgeons treat on their daily medical practice. Therefore, a large number of options have been developed for the treatment of hemorrhoids, each of them having certain indications and applications.

Hemorrhoids are normal anatomical formations of the human anal canal, playing an important role in the closure mechanism of the anal ring. The pathogenesis of hemorrhoidopathy is still not completely known, and many theories on its development have been published and debated upon. Hemorrhoids are divided in 4 stages, depending on the degree of prolapse and need for reduction. Stage 1 and 2 hemorrhoids are usually managed conservatively, whereas hemorrhoids of stage 3 and 4 often have to be treated surgically.

In 1998, Antonio Longo suggested the reduction of hemorrhoids and fixation of the prolapsing mucosa for the treatment of hemorrhoids in a technique known as PPH (Procedure for Prolapse and Hemorrhoids). When performing a PPH, a circular segment of mucosa and submucosa of the rectum is resected 2 centimeters proximal to the dentate line, using a circular stapler. For the resection, a purse-string suture is applied and tied at the 3 o'clock position. In our department, we modify the technique by applying a second suture at the 9 o'clock position. This allows us to provide a symmetrical retraction of the mucosa and submucosa into the stapler. The circular resection fixes the prolapsing mucosa and reduces the hemorrhoids. Furthermore, the staple line ligates the end branches of the superior haemorrhoidal artery, an action which reduces the blood supply to the hemorrhoids.

The procedure can be performed under general or spinal anesthesia and there is no need for prolonged hospital stay for the patient. The main advantage of the hemorrhoidopexy is the absence of postoperative pain, which was the main problem following a classical Milligan-Morgan hemorrhoidectomy. The main complications of the hemorrhoidopexy are urgency, hemorrhage and stenosis of the anal canal. The frequency of complications after PPH ranges between 6% and 31%.

In the last 10 years we performed hemorrhoidopexy in 812 patients in our department. All operations were performed under general anesthesia. The mean operating time was 14.3 minutes and the mean hospital stay 1.1 days. Postoperatively, 28 patients (3.4%) complained of mild pain for 2-9 days which was treated with plain oral analgesics. Three patients (0.3%) developed postoperative bleeding, 2 of them were treated conservatively and 1 had to be re-operated for haemostasis.

In conclusion, hemorrhoidopexy is a simple, effective, pain-free method for the treatment of mainly 3rd degree hemorrhoids with many advantages compared to the conventional hemorrhoidectomy.

INTRODUCTION

Hemorrhoidopathy is a disease known to us since ancient years. It has been mentioned in texts of ancient Greeks and Egyptians. It is believed that 20-30% of all people in the Western World will develop symptomatic hemorrhoids in a period of their lives. It is one of the commonest benign pathologies that surgeons treat on their daily medical practice. Therefore, a large number of options have been developed for the treatment of hemorrhoids, each of them having certain indications and applications (Figure1).

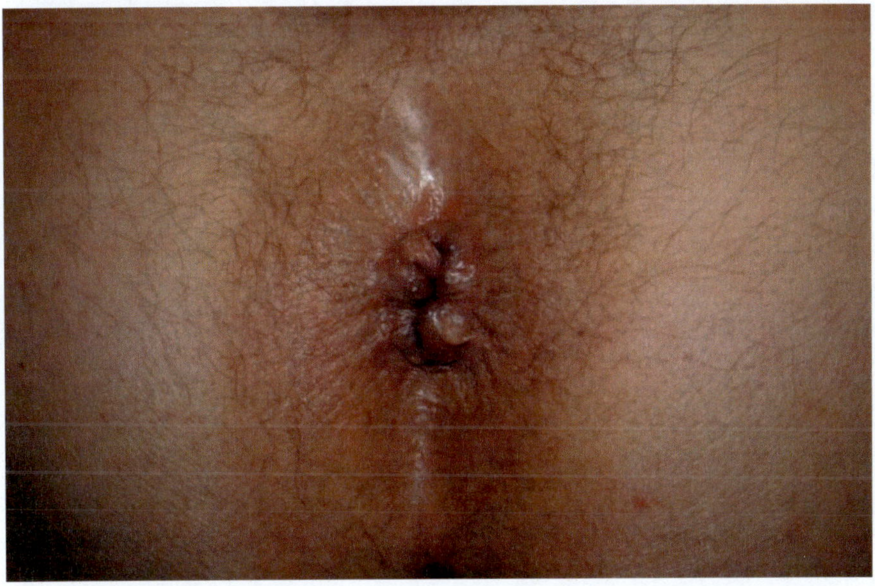

Figure 1. Hemorrhoids.

Hemorrhoids are normal anatomical formations of the human anal canal, playing an important role in the closure mechanism of the anal ring. The pathogenesis of hemorrhoidopathy is still not completely known. Many theories have been published trying to explain its development and disease course. Hemorrhoids are divided in 4 stages/degrees, depending on the degree of prolapse and need for reduction.

Stage I: Internal hemorrhoids which may bleed, but do not prolapse through the anal canal.

Stage II: Hemorrhoids that prolapse through the anal canal, usually upon defecation, but retract spontaneously.

Stage III: Hemorrhoids that require manual reduction following their prolapse.

Stage IV: Prolapsed hemorrhoids which cannot be manually reduced (Figure2).

Stage 1 and 2 hemorrhoids are usually managed conservatively, whereas hemorrhoids of stage 3 and 4 often have to be treated surgically.

The circular stapling device as a tool for the treatment of hemorrhoids was introduced by Antonio Longo in 1998, in a technique known as PPH (Procedure for Prolapse and Hemorrhoids).

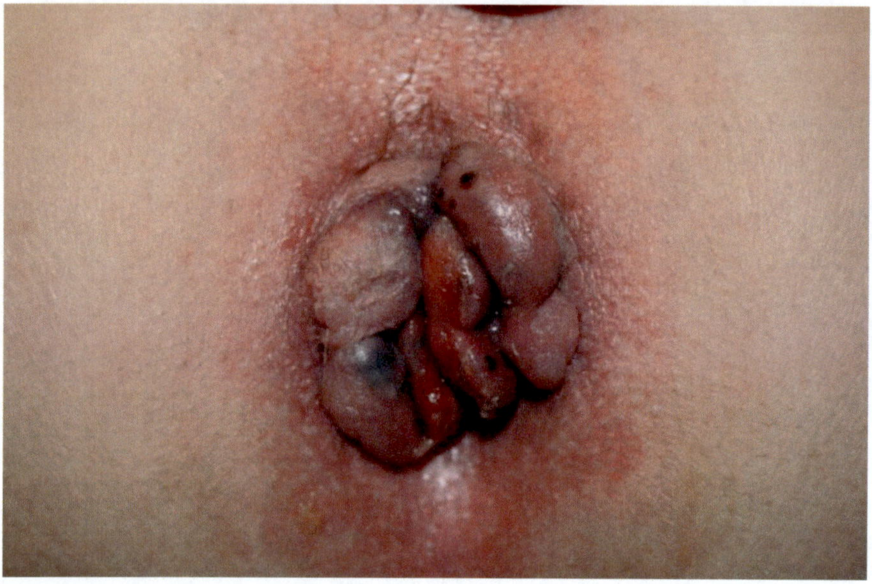

Figure 2. Prolapsed, thrombosed hemorrhoids (4th stage).

Whereas conventional surgical techniques for hemorrhoidectomy involve excision of the hemorrhoidal tissue, PPH restores the original anatomical position of the hemorrhoidal tissue by excising excess prolapsing tissue.

Since its introduction, there has been an increasing interest from surgeons across the world for PPH, mainly because of the simplicity and efficacy of the technique, the decrease of postoperative complications such as intense postoperative pain and the satisfactory long term results. By 2002, 1500 PPH procedures had already been performed in the UK. In the 5-year period between 2003 and 2008, numerous publications had appeared assessing the efficacy of the technique and comparing it to results from conventional hemorrhoidectomy procedures. International working parties published consensus positions and guidelines on the indications and use of the technique as well as recommendations and contraindications.

Aim of this chapter is to give some details on the anatomy and pathophysiology of hemorrhoids in relation to the PPH, followed by an analysis of the indications, contraindications, pre-, peri- and postoperative care, technical details and complications of the technique. In conclusion we will give an insight on our experience with this technique in Thessaloniki, Greece.

ANATOMY AND PATHOPHYSIOLOGY OF HEMORRHOIDS

Hemorrhoidal cushions are a normal component of the anal canal and are composed of vascular and connective tissue, with a rich content of collagen and elastic fibers. They are lined by simple cylindrical epithelium that is sometimes multilayered but never keratinized. They contain a high number of arteriovenous anastomoses without an interposed capillary network [1].

The speculations and pathophysiological theories for the pathogenesis of hemorrhoidal disease are various. Until today, four theories have attempted to describe this pathogenesis: the mechanical theory, the haemodynamical theory, the theory of the insufficient sphincter mechanism and the theory of Thomson.

According to the mechanical theory, the myo-fibro-elastic tissue, which supports the internal hemorrhoids, degenerates with time, usually starting during the third decade of life. This leads to a relaxation of the supporting mechanism of hemorrhoids, which makes them more mobile, whenever the intrarectal pressure tends to increase (difficult fecal evacuation or constipation). Due to that increase, the suspensory ligament and the ligament of Parks rupture, resulting to a constant prolapse of the internal hemorrhoids through the anal verge [2].

Three vascular elements participate in the hemodynamical theory of hemorrhoidal pathogenesis: arteries, veins and arteriovenous anastomoses. Internal hemorrhoids could result from retrograde venous blood flow due to increased intra-abdominal pressure (birth, difficult fecal evacuation) [3]. The dilatation of hemorrhoids could be enhanced by secondary blood stasis due to disturbed venous return (mechanical obstruction). As far as the arterial element is concerned, an increase of the visceral arterial flow, which affects the inferior mesenteric artery, could participate partially in the dilatation of the internal hemorrhoids. Based on these two vascular elements, Graham-Stewart [4] suggested that tenesmus during defecation results to an increased intraabdominal pressure and venous pressure in the hemorrhoidal plexus, resulting to the formation of hemorrhoids. In 1956, Parks suggested that the presence of hard feces in the rectum results to the obstruction and retrograde filling of the venous hemorrhoidal plexus [5]. That leads to a long term exposure of the hemorrhoids to increased pressure, resulting to a constant dilatation of the hemorrhoidal nodes.

Anorectal manometry has provided us with various types of sphincter disorders in patients suffering from hemorrhoids. The major finding is an increase of the rectal resting pressure. This increase seems to be more related to the hemorrhoids filling with blood than to an actual increase of the sphincter activity.

This spasticity disappears following a hemorrhoidectomy. Stelzner et al [6] were of the opinion that hemorrhoids, with their network of arteriovenous anastomoses, represent a closed valve, which protects the anus from gaseous and liquid incontinence.

In 1975, Thomson described a very "attractive" theory for the formation of hemorrhoids. As known, hemorrhoids appear in three main positions: left lateral, right anterior and right posterior. According to an older theory, these three positions represent the end vascular depots, being supplied by the superior hemorrhoidal artery. Thomson analyzed the three previously mentioned theories and he came to the conclusion that the hemorrhoidal nodes are nothing more than prolapsing segments of the anal canal [7]. He described "hemorrhoidal cushions", which are found in the three mentioned typical positions and are covered by a layer of fibrous tissue. Behind this layer, one finds the internal hemorrhoids. This fibro-elastic layer allows the dilatation of vessels, whenever the anal sphincter relaxes. In contrary, when the sphincter mechanism contracts it removes blood from the venules, which remain almost empty.

INDICATIONS

As far as the indications for the hemorrhoidopexy are concerned, there have been numerous consensus meetings and discussions in order to highlight the patient cases where the mentioned technique can and should be applied. In 2003, a consensus meeting by an international expert working party on stapled hemorrhoidopexy identified the indications for the use of that technique [8]. According to that meeting, the following are the accepted indications for a hemorrhoidopexy:

- Failure to alleviate hemorrhoidal symptoms by other methods (such as rubber band ligation)
- Selected prolapsing hemorrhoids with spontaneous reduction (Grade II)
- Prolapsing hemorrhoids requiring manual reduction (Grade III)
- Uncomplicated hemorrhoids, irreducible by the patient but reducible at surgery (Grade IV).

In 2006, the Italian Society of Colorectal Surgery concurred that, as far as the indications for a hemorrhoidopexy are concerned, these must certainly include [9]:

- repeated bleeding episodes which are difficult to control pharmacologically
- external prolapse of the hemorrhoidal tissue
- a tendency to repeated hemorrhoidal thrombosis

It is important to mention that, in case of rectal bleeding, other causes of bleeding should be excluded before proceeding to surgical management of the hemorrhoids. Furthermore, severe anaemia secondary to hemorrhoidal bleeding should never be an indication for surgery even in high-risk patients.

Contra-Indications

The hemorrhoidopexy is a relatively safe technique for the treatment of hemorrhoids, as long as it is performed by trained surgeons, aware of the steps of that procedure. Nevertheless, there are cases where the hemorrhoidopexy should not be applied as a treatment option for hemorrhoids. The 2003 consensus meeting on the stapled hemorrhoidopexy procedure concluded to the following conditions as contra-indications for the procedure [8]:

- abscess
- gangrene
- anal stenosis
- full-thickness rectal prolapse

It is important to know that the performance of a stapled hemorrhoidopexy in the presence of gangrenous or infected tissue is absolutely contraindicated. The reason for the latter is, on one hand, that the hemorrhoidopexy does not remove the septic source and on the other hand the fact that opening additional tissue planes may expose the patient to pelvic sepsis and to the possibility of Fournier's gangrene.

The presence of anal stenosis makes the insertion of the anal dilator difficult, risking damage to the anoderm or the mucosa. Finally, there is no evidence that the procedure successfully treats full-thickness prolapse [8].

In patients with coagulation deficiencies, using the circular stapler has shown positive results in published series, in contrary to traditional hemorrhoidectomy which is associated with an increased bleeding risk. Nevertheless, patients under warfarin sodium treatment should have it replaced with a low molecular weight heparin before surgery and for the first postoperative week [10].

Pregnancy often exacerbates hemorrhoids due to its association with increased pelvic pressure and constipation. Even though conservative treatment should be the treatment of choice, hemorrhoidectomy has been performed in pregnant patients with success. No published studies have assessed the specific success rate of hemorrhoidopexy in these situations [11].

Pre-Operative Investigations and Anesthesia

No special or specific preoperative investigations are required for a patient who is planned to undergo a stapled hemorrhoidopexy. The pre-operative work-up is similar to that of a patient undergoing a conventional hemorrhoidectomy. Depending on the medical condition of the patient and any associated medical problems, one should have general laboratory results of the patient, including full blood count, renal function and electrolytes. The procedure can be performed as a day-case procedure, which means that the patient can be admitted to the hospital on the day of the operation. Bowel preparation usually includes a rectal enema two hours prior to the operation. It is suggested that the patient should receive one shot of a 2nd generation cephalosporin and metronidazole [12].

The procedure can be performed under local, epidural or general anesthesia. The choice lies upon the surgeon and the anesthetist performing the procedure. In our institution, we prefer general anaesthesia when performing a PPH. There is general consensus that if local anesthesia is elected, conscious sedation should be used. The suture placements can cause discomfort which may be unsuccessfully controlled by local anesthetics alone [13].

Technique

Positioning of the patient depends on the surgeon. Advantages and disadvantages have been found with both the lithotomy and the prone/jackknife position. Surgeons tend to prefer the position they are comfortable with when performing a conventional hemorrhoidectomy.

The PPH set includes the following instruments (Figure 3):

- Circular stapler of 33 mm diameter

- Transparent circular anal dilator
- Anoscope for the purse-string suture
- Suture threader

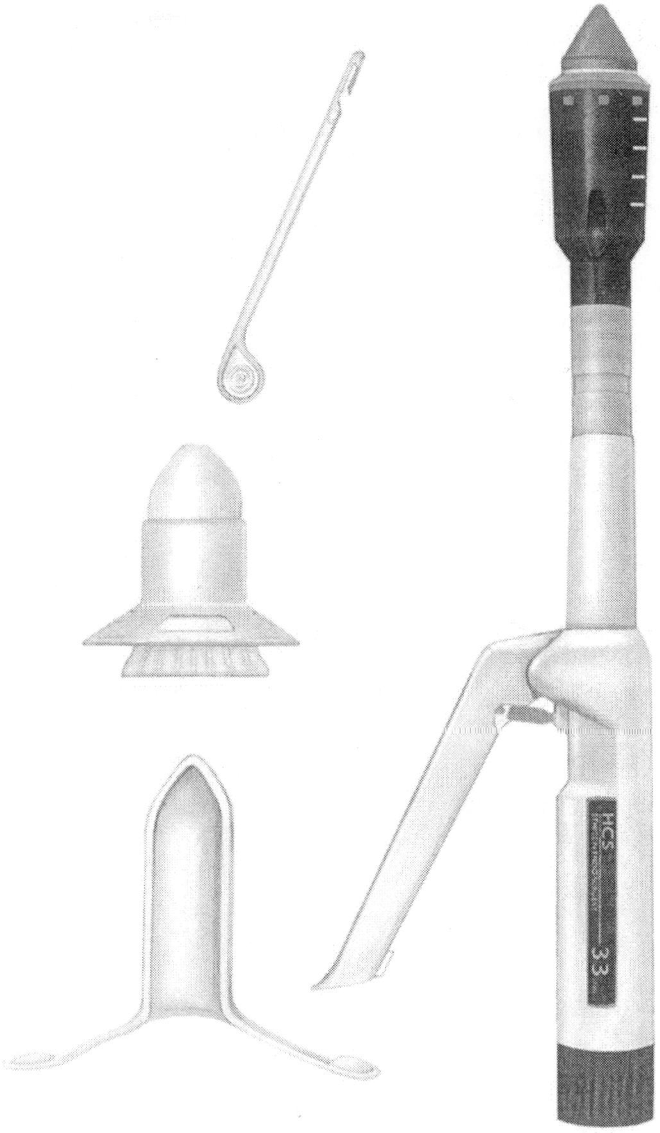

Figure 3. The PPH instrumentarium.

All instruments are specifically designed for the hemorrhoidopexy. The operation is performed as described in the next steps:

The anodermal line is grasped with 3 Duvall graspers in 3 spots where the degree of prolapse is smaller and the anoderm is turned slightly outwards.

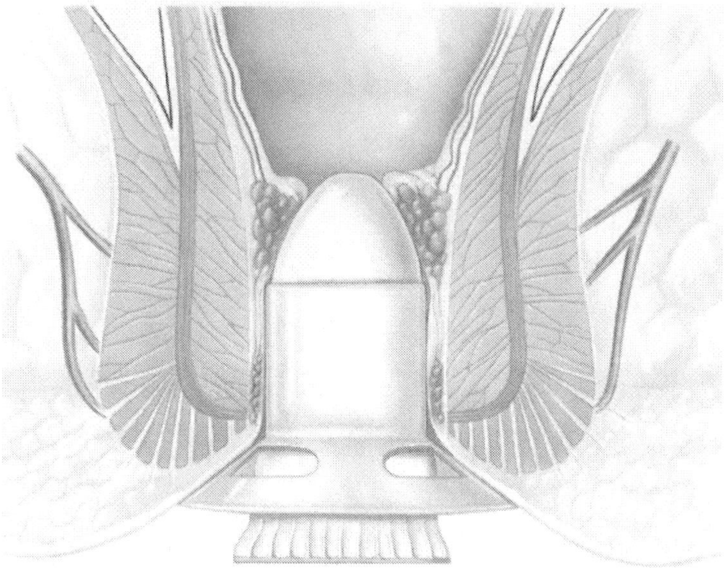

Figure 4. Insertion of the anal dilator

At first, the anal dilator is inserted in the anus, well lubricated and without sphincter stretch (Figure 4). Counter traction should be applied to the skin to facilitate the insertion. If stenosis precludes the passage, the procedure should be aborted. It is necessary that the whole dilator is inserted in the rectum. The insertion of the dilator reduces the anoderm prolapse. After removal of the obturator, the prolapsing mucosa enters the dilator lumen. The instrument transparency allows visibility of the dentate line. The anal dilator is anchored to the skin by means of a heavy suture in the 3, 6, 9 and 12 o'clock positions (Figure5).

Following that, the anoscope is inserted through the dilator. This instrument will longitudinally hold the prolapsing mucosa while leaving an opening of 90 degrees, which can easily accommodate a suture which would include mucosa and submucosa (Figure 6). Clockwise rotation of the anoscope allows consecutive stitches of mucosa and submucosa, resulting in a purse-string suture of the whole canal (Figure 7). That purse-string suture is placed 2 cm above the apex of the hemorrhoids (3-4 cm from the dentate line) with a 2/0 monofilament nylon suture on a 26mm round-bodied needle (Figure 6). The suture steps need to be many and short (3-4 mm) instead of few large ones.

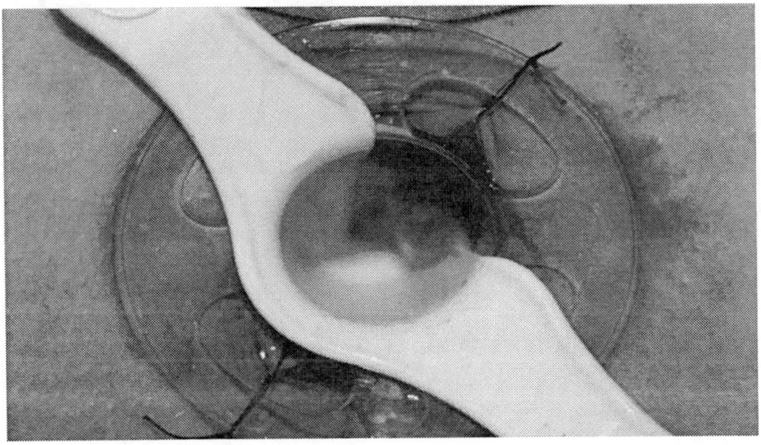

Figure 5. Anchoring of the dilator to the skin.

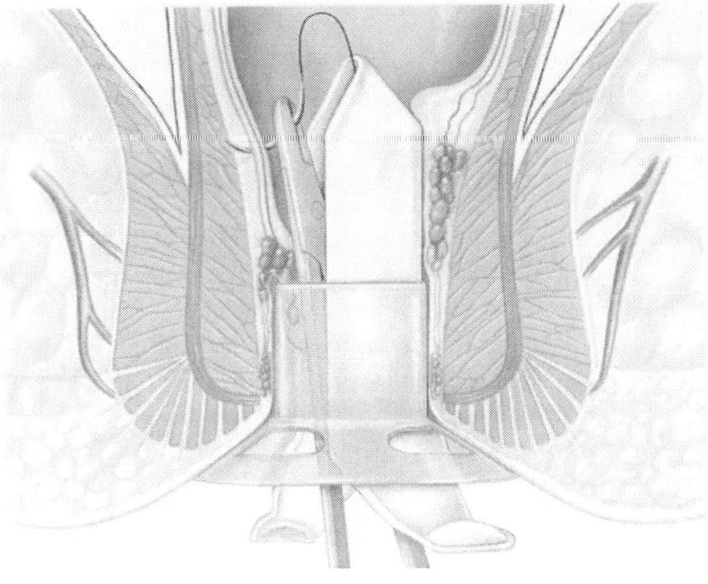

Figure 6. Mucosa-submucosa suture through the anoscope opening.

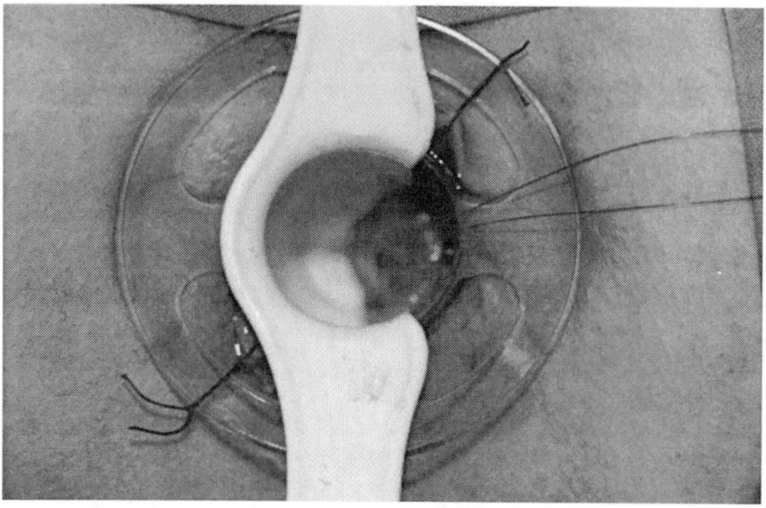

Figure 7. Purse-string suture at 3 o'clock position (lithotomy).

Right-handed surgeons usually begin the purse-string suture at the 3 o'clock position and proceed in a clockwise manner, whereas left-handed surgeons might prefer beginning at the 9 o'clock position and proceed anticlockwise.

As a next step, the anoscope is removed. In case of asymmetrical prolapse of the mucosa and the hemorrhoids, it is possible to create two "half-purse-string" sutures. The distance between these two sutures depends on the prolapse asymmetry. In female patients, it is necessary to perform a digital vaginal examination to ensure that the posterior vaginal wall has not accidentally been included in the purse string suture.

The circular stapler head is opened fully and inserted via the dilator in order for the head to pass proximally to the purse-string suture (Figure 8). The suture is then tied at the neck of the circular stapler. The suture ends are pulled through the lateral stapler channels with the help of the suture threader (Figure 9). The suture ends are then tied externally and pulled with a grasper, providing the appropriate tension in order for the mucosal segment that will be excised to be pulled between the head and the base of the circular stapler (Figure 10). Before closing and firing the stapler, it is of particular importance that the axis of the circular stapler is the same as the longitudinal axis of the anal canal. The circular stapler is then closed, while maintaining adequate tension on the purse string, and fired (Figure 11,12). This cuts and sutures the mucosa 2 cm proximal to the dentate line. Once again, in female patients the vaginal wall is assessed in order to ensure that it is not incorporated in the resection strip.

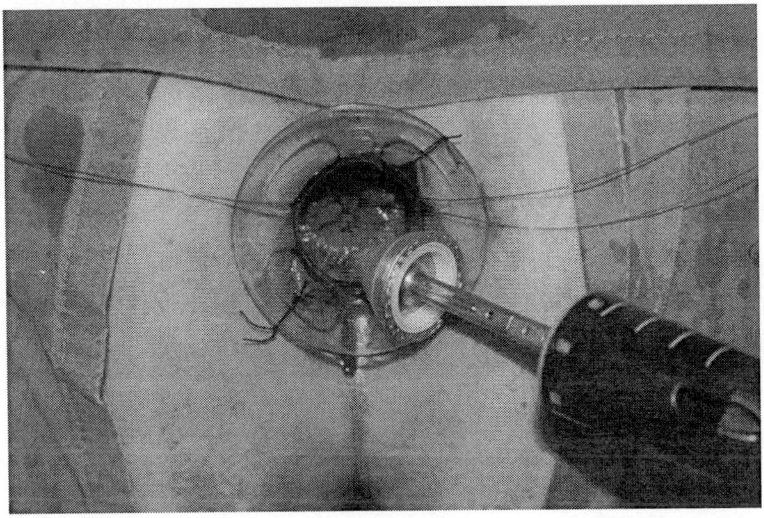

Figure 8. Insertion of the stapler (fully opened).

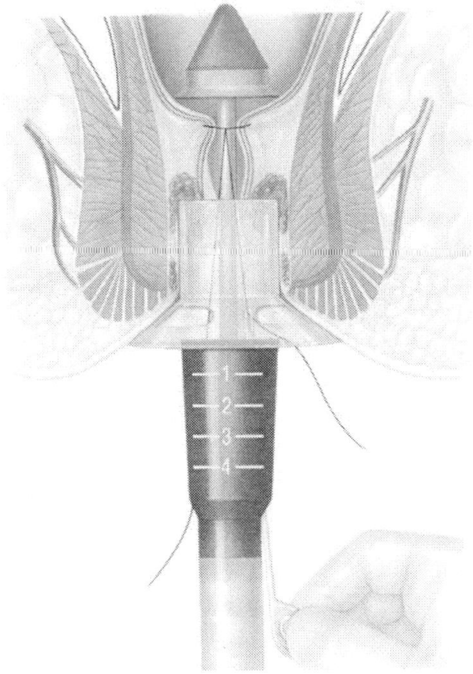

Figure 9. Suture threader pulling the suture ends through the lateral channels.

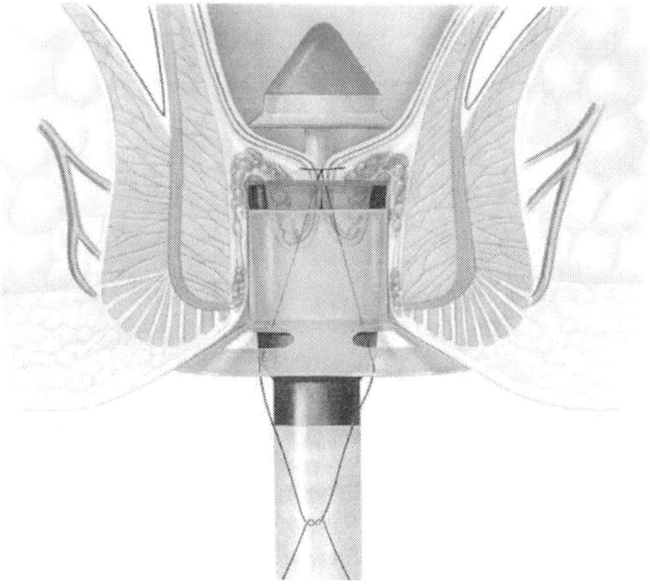

Figure 10. Suture tension for the mucosa traction in the stapler.

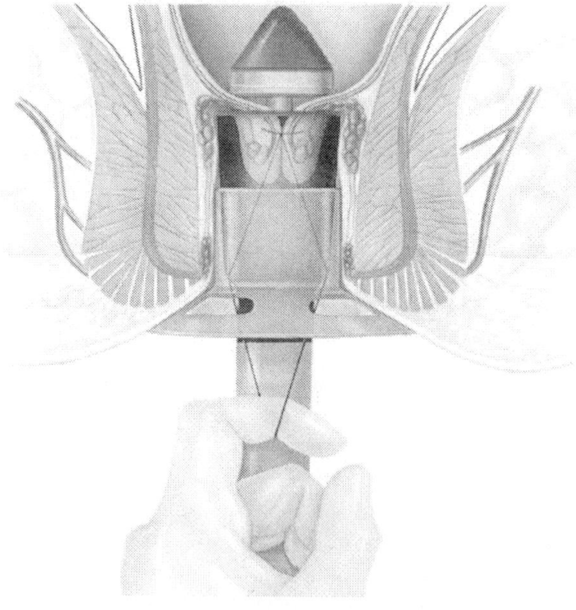

Figure 11. Closure of the stapler under tension of the mucosa.

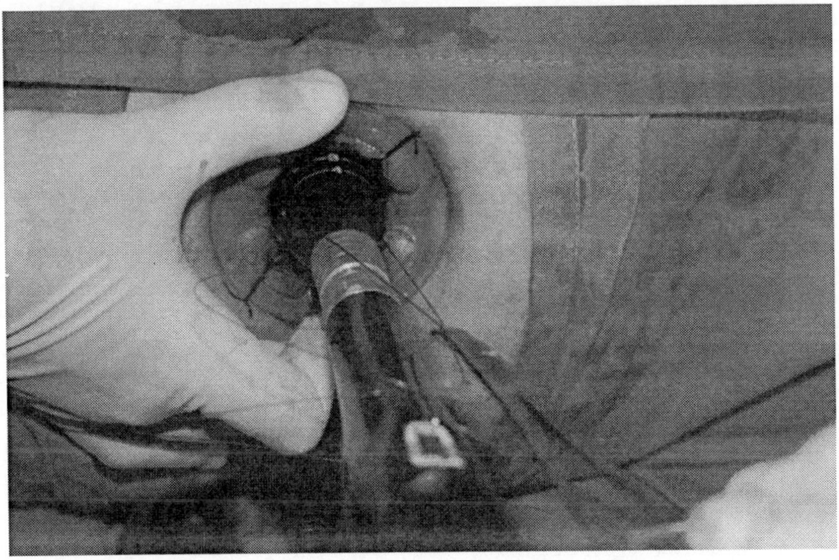

Figure 12. Maintaining longitudinal axis of stapler and anal canal, before firing.

The circular stapler is kept closed for 60 seconds to strengthen anastomotic haemostasis. Following that, the stapler is opened and removed carefully. The staple line ligates the end branches of the superior haemorrhoidal artery, an action which reduces the blood supply to the hemorrhoids and assists in their reduction (Figure 13).

At the end, the staple line is inspected for possible bleeding points with the help of the anoscope. Haemostasis can be achieved with the help of pressure, coagulation or suturing with absorbable material.

In cases where the mucosal prolapse is larger than 3 cm, it is advisable that a second purse string suture is applied 2 cm proximal to the first one. Large skin tags can be excised with the help of diathermy.

After completion, the reduction of the prolapsing mucosa and hemorrhoids is already visible. The operation is completed with anal dressing or gauze according to surgeon's preference.

The instrumentarium of the PPH set ensures correct placement of the purse-string suture at the base of the hemorrhoidal nodes. The anal dilator keeps the sphincter relaxed and allows the atraumatic placement of the purse-string suture. The purse-string anoscope helps the distance measurement between the dentate line and the suture and simplifies its placement. The circular stapler is very ergonomic and allows the resection of large mucosal prolapse.

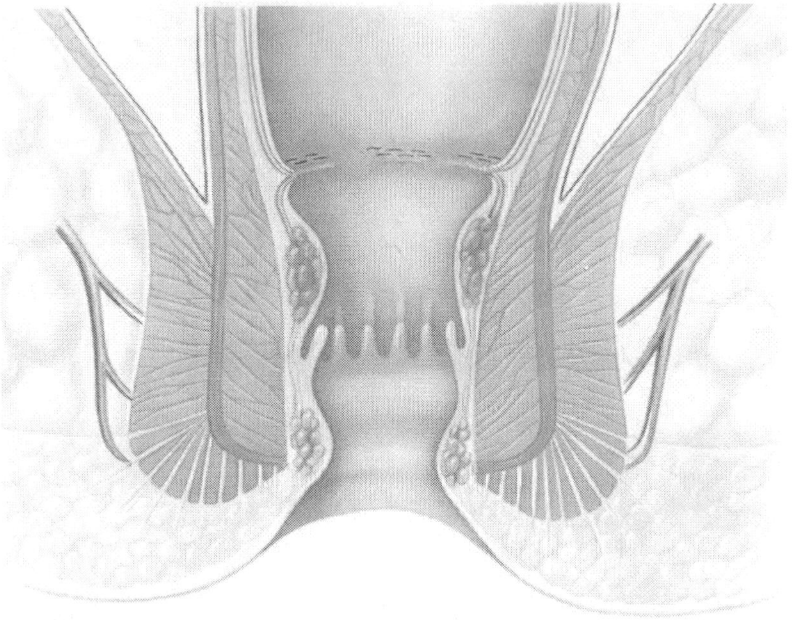

Figure 13. Completed hemorrhoidopexy.

The fact that the resection can be adjusted by externally pulling on the suture ends and by adjusting the level of the purse-string suture is very important in improving the results of this technique.

Technique Modification

After performing a PPH on around 140 patients, we observed that the mucosal sleeve that was removed with the stapler was asymmetric, meaning that its width wasn't the same at the whole length of the strip. The reason for that was that the tension on the purse string suture was higher towards the side where the suture was tied (usually the 3 'clock position). Therefore, the mucosal staple line wasn't straight in these patients. This means that the reduction of some of the hemorrhoidal nodes would be incomplete with a higher risk of hemorrhoidal recurrence at these points. Whenever though we had a large rectal prolapse and applied two different purse string sutures, the first of which was tied at the 3 o'clock position and the second at the 9 o'clock position, the resected sleeve was symmetric, meaning of equal width at its whole length.

That observation lead us to always applying an additional simple suture parallel to the purse string suture at the 9 o'clock position, which was tied. The purse string was tied at the 3 o'clock position as usual (Figure 14,15). The ends of the purse string suture and the additional suture were pulled through the two lateral channels in the head of the stapler with the help of the suture threader. By applying traction simultaneously on these two ends, the mucosal traction was symmetrical at the whole length of the mucosal strip while firing the stapler. The sleeve that was removed had the same width at its whole length.

We believe that this modification allows the symmetrical reduction of all hemorrhoids, therefore improving the hemorrhoidopexy technique and minimizing the risk of recurrence.

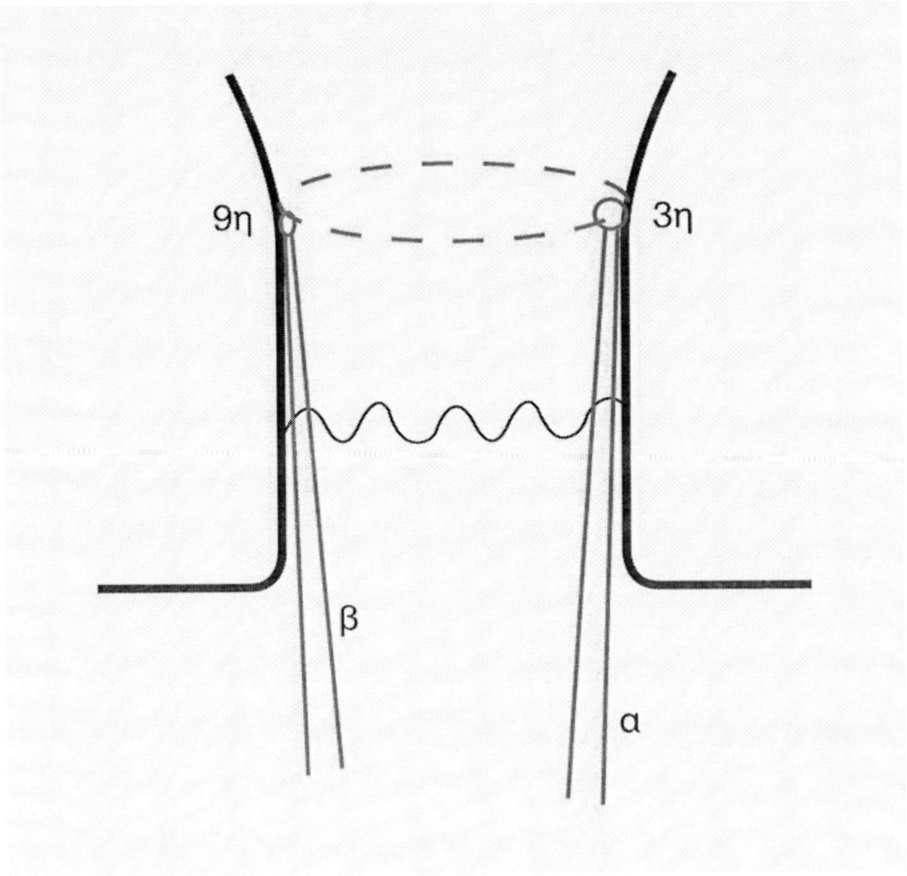

Figure 14. Technique modification (Kanellos et al).

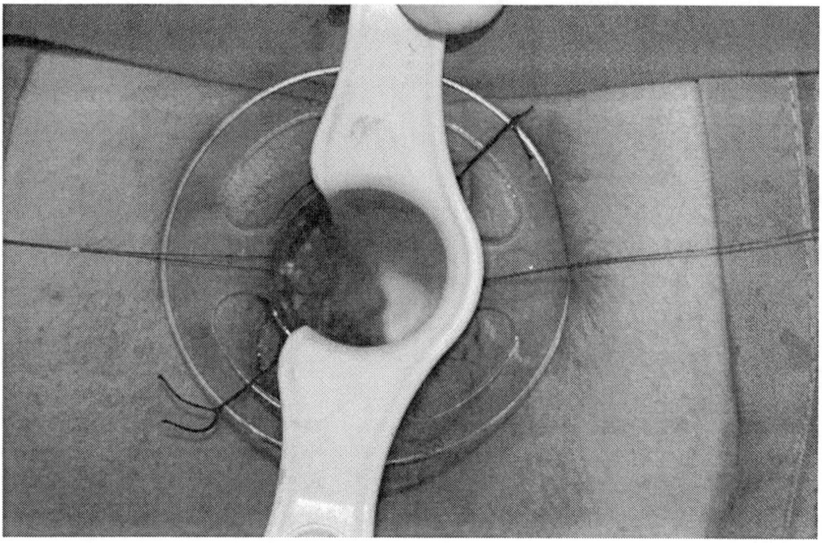

Figure 15. Purse string suture at 3 o'clock position with additional 9 o'clock position single suture.

POSTOPERATIVE CARE

Postoperative analgesia in the form of oral analgesia is sometimes required. Urinary retention is an occasional problem in male patients. They should be encouraged to drink good amounts of water on the afternoon of the operation day and try to urinate. It is safe to discharge the patient on the evening of the operation day or on the first postoperative day. Patients should be informed of the possibility of small amounts of rectal blood during the first postoperative days. They should be encouraged to return to their normal daily activity as soon as possible. Patients need to be alerted that the appearance of intense postoperative pain, fever, urinary retention or inability to pass gas/faeces needs to be reported to the surgeon promptly, as these could be signs of perineal infection [14, 15].

Overall, the risk of postoperative pain and complications is low, when the technique is applied correctly. The esthetic results are very satisfactory.

MANAGING ASSOCIATED CONDITIONS

It is not uncommon for hemorrhoids to co-exist with other pathologies or conditions of the anus. The commonest are:

- Anal skin tags (Figure 16)
- Anal fissure (Figure 17)
- Anal fistula
- Thrombosis
- Pre-existing sphincter injury
- Excessive rectal mucosal prolapse
- Anal intercourse

Anal skin tags can be assessed intraoperatively and can be resected at the same time, as long as that resection does not increase the infection risk of the operative area.

Anal fissure is traditionally managed at the time of conventional hemorrhoidectomy by sphincterotomy at the typical 3 o'clock position. During hemorrhoidopexy, the fissure can also be managed at the same time. We operated on 97 patients with co-existing hemorrhoids and chronic anal fissure, resistant to conservative therapy. The anal fissure was managed first with a lateral internal sphincterotomy at the 3 o'clock position, followed by a hemorrhoidopexy with a circular stapler (Figure 18). Performing the sphincterotomy in the beginning makes the procedure easier, because the anatomy of the area is not yet disturbed. Moreover, the application of the anal dilator for the insertion of the stapler applies pressure on the sphincterotomy area, improving haemostasis. All fissures in our patient series healed in a period of four weeks. Most patients were satisfied with the operation results, apart from 15 patients (15%) who developed some degree of sphincter incontinence, which gradually improved in the 6-8 weeks to follow. During postoperative follow-up, no patient presented with hemorrhoid or fissure recurrence [16].

Anal fistulas, especially low-lying ones, can be successfully treated at the same time as the hemorrhoids. An experienced surgeon can assess the fistula and decide whether it is safe to proceed to a hemorrhoidopexy after laying open the fistula, as this is going to create an open wound which could lead to area infection and septic complications (Figure 19) [8].

Acute hemorrhoidal thrombosis is a concern if a stapled hemorrhoidopexy is to be performed (Figure 2). It is recommended that the thrombotic area is incised and removed if a hemorrhoidopexy is to be undertaken.

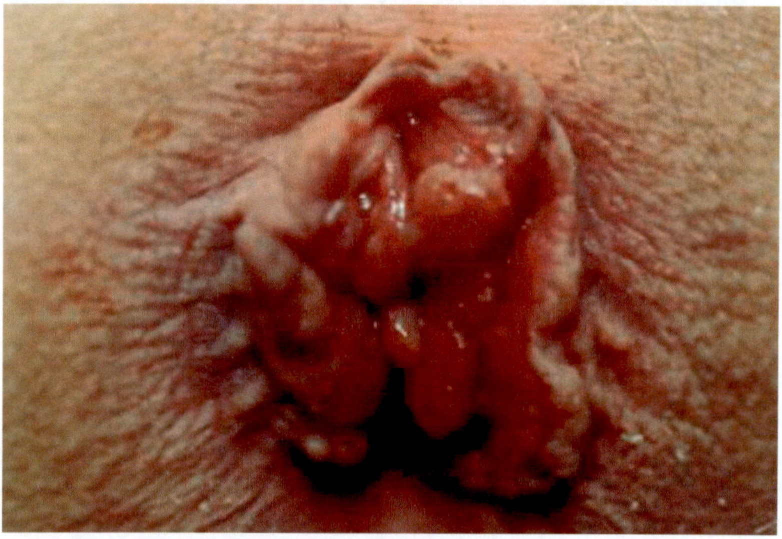

Figure 16. Anal skin tags.

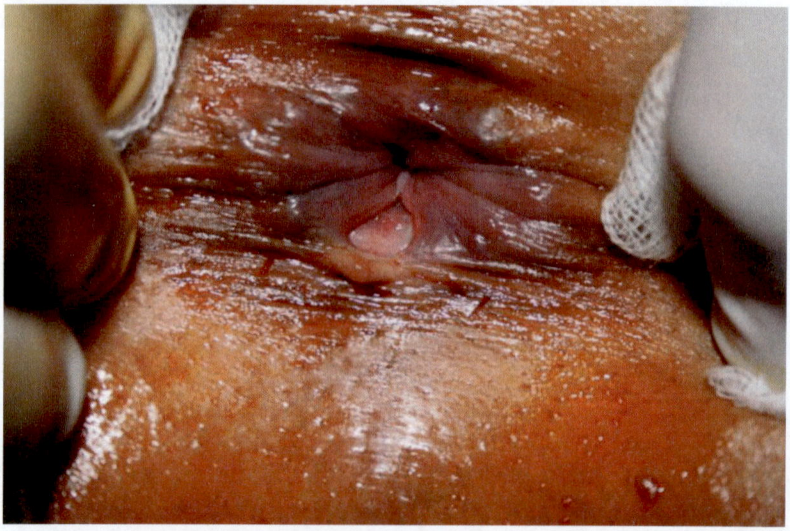

Figure 17. Anal fissure.

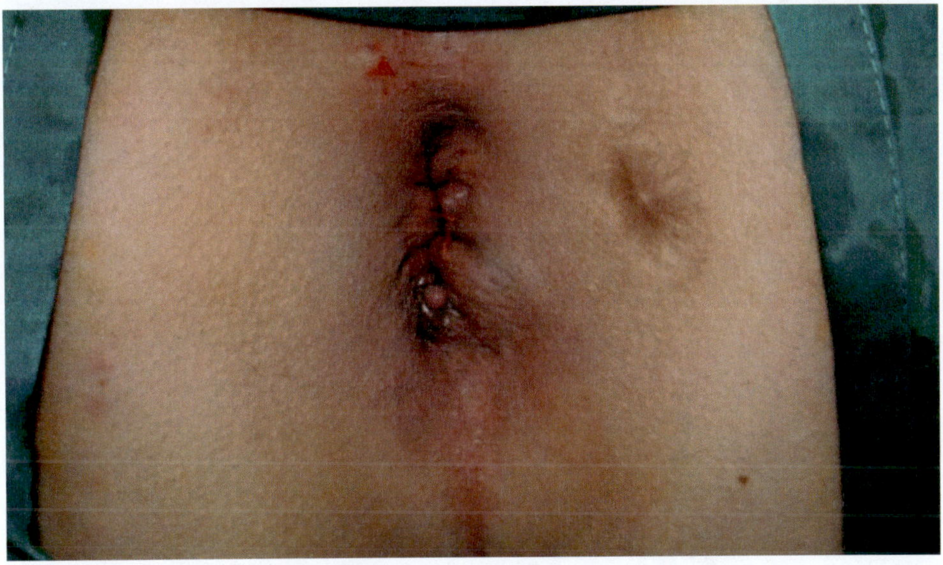

Figure 18. Combined internal sphincterotomy with PPH.

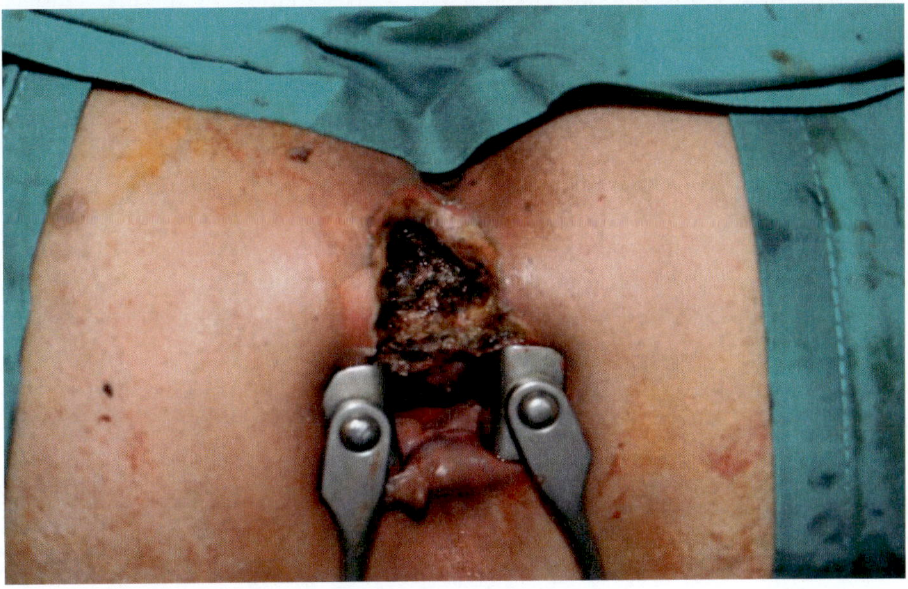

Figure 19. Laid-open anal fistula combined with PPH.

Pre-existing sphincter injury or anal incontinence is to be seriously considered when a PPH is planned. The reason for that is that the hemorrhoidopexy requires the insertion of a relatively large anal dilator. The stretch associated with that insertion can lead to further damage of the sphincter mechanism, resulting to bowel control impairment.

Rectal mucosal prolapse can be successfully treated along with the hemorrhoids when performing a hemorrhoidopexy. In case of excessive prolapse, it may be difficult to fully insert the stapler or to encompass all tissue necessary. Full-thickness rectal prolapse cannot be treated successfully with a hemorrhoidopexy [8].

Anal intercourse needs to be addressed to patients undergoing hemorrhoidopexy. Even though the staples slough out or ultimately become completely buried within the mucosa and submucosa, there is a small risk of penile injury during anal intercourse in the first months after a hemorrhoidopexy.

Postoperative Complications

The major complications that have been reported with the classical hemorrhoidectomy are bleeding, anal stenosis and anal fissure. Minor complications include pain, urinary retention, urinary tract infections, perineal haematoma or abscess, urgency/tenesmus, anal pruritus, anal fistulas and gas or faecal incontinence. The commonest late complication is the recurrence. The complications following a hemorrhoidopexy are similar to the ones after a classical hemorrhoidectomy, while additional ones that have been reported include hemorrhoidal thrombosis, anastomotic leak leading to pelvic sepsis, rectal obstruction, **retrorectal haematomas and Fournier's gangrene** [17].

The complication rate after hemorrhoidopexy ranges from 6% to 31% [14]. Some published studies tend to correlate the complication rate with the learning curve of the surgeon. Nevertheless, a 2002 multi-center trial from Italy on 1107 patients from 20 different centers showed that this was not the case [18]. Most complications occurred on surgeons who had already performed at least 25 procedures. In this particular study the complication rate was 15% (164/1107). Early complications (1st postoperative week) included pain in 5% of patients, bleeding in 4.2%, thrombosis in 2.3%, urinary retention in 1.5% and anastomotic leak in 0.5%. The most frequent late complications were hemorrhoid recurrence in 2.3% and stenosis in 0.8% of the patients.

In 2005, the Association of Coloproctology of Great Britain and Ireland set up an online electronic database to audit the indications and outcomes for patients undergoing a PPH procedure [19]. 61 surgeons were included in this audit, with a total of 695 patients. 57.1% of these patients had grade III or IV hemorrhoids. In this audit, 75 patients (10.8%) presented with early complications. The commonest were bleeding in 3% and urinary retention in 3.5% of the patients. At 6 week follow-up, 90.1% of patients were pain free. The commonest problems at follow-up were bleeding in 5.9%, urgency in 2.7% and pain in 1.7% of the patients.

The main advantage of the hemorrhoidopexy compared to classical hemorrhoidectomy is the absence of postoperative pain. As the anal wall is innervated by sympathetic and parasympathetic fibers, the excision of a circular sleeve of the rectal mucosa should be painless. In order for that to happen, the application of the purse-string suture should be 2 cm proximal to the base of the hemorrhoids. If the suturing finds place close to the dentate line then there is a high probability of postoperative pain. Postoperative pain or discomfort for a few days can also be due to intense stretch of the sphincter mechanism during the operation. If extreme dilation of the anal canal is avoided and the purse string is applied to the correct position, the appearance of postoperative pain is unusual. Another parameter that was assessed was the inclusion of muscle fibers in the dissected mucosal ring. In a group of 94 patients, the removed specimens underwent histological examination [18]. In 65 cases where the specimen did not include muscle fibers, postoperative pain presented in 26% of patients, whereas when the specimens included muscle fibers, 66% of patients developed postoperative pain. Even though pain can appear when muscle fibers are not dissected, the chances of postoperative pain are higher when the muscle is damaged. Therefore, it is important that the purse-string suture extends to the mucosa and submucosa only, and does not include muscular layers.

As far as the return to daily activities is concerned, the comparison between hemorrhoidopexy and classical hemorrhoidectomy is doubtful [20]. Even though less postoperative pain and faster wound healing would make someone expect patients who underwent hemorrhoidopexy to return to their daily activities faster, this is not the case. The latter depends on various socioeconomic factors, and should therefore not be used as a statistical comparison parameter for the outcome of the two techniques.

Bleeding is the second commonest early complication after a hemorrhoidopexy. The circular stapler clips do not always achieve complete haemostasis even when the purse-string suture is applied correctly. More often, the suture is too deep in the rectal wall resulting to the inclusion of a very thick ring of tissue in the staple line of the stapler. A practical solution for added haemostasis is to keep the stapler closed after firing for at least 60 seconds, applying pressure to the suture line. The frequency of immediate bleeding after removing the stapler ranges between 4% and 60% [8,17,18]. It is important to reinsert the anoscope after completing the procedure and to carefully inspect the suture line for bleeding spots. If bleeding is observed, this can be controlled with either the application of adrenaline solution (1:200000) or with the application of haemostatic sutures. In the previously mentioned study by Ravo et al [18], a group of 46 patients with postoperative bleeding were controlled with additional suturing in 24%, the insertion of a Folley catheter in 15% and adrenaline application in 7%. In the remaining 53% of patients, the bleeding stopped automatically without any intervention.

Urinary retention is reported in 1.5% of patients undergoing hemorrhoidopexy under general anesthesia [21]. When the procedure is performed under local anesthesia, this percentage seems to increase. In a study of 59 patients who underwent PPH under local anesthetic, 27% developed urinary retention [22]. The authors believe that this is due to the infiltration of the urinary bladder wall and its nerve endings by local anesthetic, resulting to temporary function loss.

Another less common early complication is the appearance of a perineal haematoma, that can be managed conservatively or by external drainage if necessary.

Urgency was not given the appropriate attention when the method started being used. Today, bibliographic evidence and our personal experience make us aware that 20-35% of patients will develop urgency/tenesmus after a PPH. It usually settles 2-4 weeks after the procedure. Spasmolytics such as Mebeverine Hydrochloride can be used conservatively for the management of urgency.

Anal fissures result when the mucosal ring incorporated in the stapler is too thick, resulting in high tension at the edge of the mucosa. This may cause the mucosa to tear and lead to the creation of a fissure. The only solution is the complete removal of the clips, in order for the mucosal tension to disappear.

Gas or fecal incontinence has been reported in some studies. It is usually temporary incontinence (Grade I or II) due to the intra-operative mechanical stretch of the sphincter mechanism. A stapler of smaller diameter might be the solution to that complication [8,18].

Anastomotic leakage is a rare complication, which can lead to severe sepsis. In a 2000 study by Herold and Kirsch [23], 4635 patients who underwent hemorrhoidopexy in 224 German hospitals were assessed. 3 cases of rectal perforation were reported (two needing temporary defunctioning and one a permanent colostomy), one case of complete rectal obstruction, one case of a large retrorectal haematoma and one case of Fournier's gangrene resulting to death. Such severe complications have also been reported in other studies but it is relatively simple to avoid them, as long as one pays attention to the correct application of the purse-string suture [24]. It should involve only part of the bowel wall and the anastomosis should incorporate mucosa and submucosa only. When suspicious signs of postoperative sepsis are present, such as high fever, pain, urinary or fecal retention, patients should undergo radiological studies with plain radiographs or abdominal computed tomography. The presence of air in the pelvis is a serious sign of a possible pelvic or retroperitoneal infection. The immediate onset of antibiotics can possibly limit the infection spread and could avoid the necessity of a reoperation.

The commonest late complication after a hemorrhoidopexy is the recurrence of the hemorrhoids. In a multicenter study by Ravo et al [18], 2.3% of 1107 patients developed recurrence after a PPH. The authors report that, when a patient complains of hemorrhoidal symptoms after a hemorrhoidopexy, these symptoms should not be referred to as a recurrence. In reality, the hemorrhoids were never removed. Recurrence refers to the reappearance of symptoms similar to the ones that lead the patient to the surgeon the first time. In the previously reported study, 40% of patients that presented with recurrence were treated with rubber band ligation and 32% with a Milligan-Morgan hemorrhoidectomy [18]. In a study assessing the long-term results of PPH for 3rd degree hemorrhoids published in 2006, recurrence occurred in 8 out of 126 patients (6.3%) over a follow-up period of 5 years [17]. One year later, the same research team assessed the long-term results of PPH for 4th degree hemorrhoids over a follow-up time period of 6 years, and found the recurrence rate to be 58.9% (33 out of 56 patients) [14]. Based on these results and on our experience, we suggest that the hemorrhoidopexy using PPH is ideally indicated for 3rd degree hemorrhoids and not for 4th degree ones. We believe that 4th degree hemorrhoids should be managed with a Milligan-Morgan hemorrhoidectomy. It is important to note that, in case of a hemorrhoidal recurrence, the hemorrhoidopexy using PPH can be repeated, in a similar manner as the first time.

Less common late complications after PPH include anal stenosis (which can be managed with manual dilatations), the creation of a mucosal diaphragm (requiring dissection), while there have been reports of rectal intussusception, which was managed with rectopexy.

Our Experience

In the last 10 years we performed hemorrhoidopexy on 812 patients in Thessaloniki, Greece. All operations were performed under general anesthesia. The mean operating time was 14.3 minutes and the mean hospital stay 1.1 days. Postoperatively, 28 patients (3.4%) complained of mild pain for 2-9 days which was treated with oral analgesia. 28 patients (3.4%) developed urinary retention in the postoperative period, which was managed with the insertion of a urinary catheter. Three patients (0.3%) developed postoperative bleeding, 2 of them were treated conservatively and 1 had to be re-operated for haemostasis. Urgency appeared in 216 patients (26.6%) for a period of 2-4 weeks, and it settled on its own with conservative support by spasmolytics.

Conclusion

The hemorrhoidopexy using PPH has many advantages compared to the conventional hemorrhoidectomy, the most important being the absence of postoperative pain. Patients can be treated as day-cases, and the procedure has a low rate of post-operative complications. In the hands of an experienced surgeon, hemorrhoidopexy with PPH is a simple, safe and effective method for the treatment of mainly 3rd degree hemorrhoids.

Acknowledgements

Images 3, 4, 6, 9-11, 13 are courtesy of Johnson and Johnson Hellas. Images 1, 2, 5, 7, 8, 12, 14-19 belong to the private collection of Prof. Ioannis Kanellos.

References

[1] Hulme-Moir M, Bartolo DC. Disorders of the anorectum. *Gastroenterol. Clin. North Am.* 2001; 30: 183-197.

[2] Hass PA, Fox TA, Haas GP. The pathogenesis of hemorrhoids. *Dis. Colon Rectum.* 1984; 27: 442-450.

[3] Mazier WP. Hemorrhoids, fissures and pruritus ani. *Surg. Clin. North Am.* 1994; 74: 1977-1992.

[4] Graham-Stewart CW. What causes hemorrhoids? A new theory of etiology. *Dis. Colon Rectum* 1963; 6: 333-334.

[5] Parks AG. Surgical treatment of hemorrhoids. *Br. J. Surg.* 1956; 43: 337.

[6] Stelzner F, Staubesand J, Machleidt. Das corpus cavernosum recti. *Arch. Klin. Chir.* (Berlin) 1982; 299-302.

[7] Thomson WBF. The nature of hemorrhoids. *Br. J. Surg.* 1975; 62: 542-52.

[8] Corman ML, Gravie JF, Hager T, Loudon MA, Mascagni D, Nystrom PO, Seow-Choen F, Abcarian H, Marcello P, Weiss E, Longo A. Stapled hemorrhoidopexy: a consensus position paper by an international working party – indications, contra-indications and technique. *Colorectal Dis.* 2003; 5: 304-310.

[9] Altomare DF, Roveran A, Pecorella G, Gaj F, Stortini E. The treatment of hemorrhoids: guidelines of the Italian Society of Colo-Rectal Surgery. *Tech. Coloproctol.* 2006; 10: 181-186.

[10] Lawes DA, Palazzo FF, Clifton MA. The use of Ligasure hemorrhoidectomy in patients taking oral anticoagulation therapy. *Colorectal Dis.* 2003; 6: 111-112.

[11] Saleeby RG, Rosen L, Stasik SJ, Riether RD, Sheets J, Khubchandani IT. Haemorrhoidectomy during pregnancy: risk or relief? *Dis. Colon Rectum.* 1991; 34: 260-261.

[12] Goulimaris I, Kanellos I, Christoforidis E, Mantzoros I, Odisseos Ch, Betsis D. Stapled hemorrhoidectomy compared with Milligan-Morgan excision for the treatment of prolapsing hemorrhoids. *Eur. J. Surg.* 2002; 168: 621-625.

[13] Shalaby R, Desoky A. Randomized clinical trial of stapled versus Milligan-Morgan hemorrhoidectomy. *Br. J. Surg.* 2001; 88: 1049-1053.

[14] Zacharakis E, Kanellos D, Pramateftakis MG, Kanellos I, Angelopoulos S, Mantzoros I, Betsis D. Long-term results after stapled haemorrhoidopexy for fourth-degree haemorrhoids: a prospective study with median follow-up of 6 years. *Tech. Coloproctol.* 2007; 11: 144-147.

[15] Mehigan BJ, Monson JTR, Hartley JE. Stapling procedure for haemorrhoids versus Milligan-Morgan haemorrhoidectomy: randomized controlled trial. *Lancet* 2000; 355: 782-785.

[16] Kanellos I, Angelopoulos S, Zacharakis E, Kanellos D, Pramateftakis MG, Blouhos K, Betsis D. Stapled haemorrhoidopexy for haemorrhoids in combination with lateral internal sphincterotomy for fissure-in-ano. *Eur. Surg. Res.* 2005; 37: 317-320.

[17] Kanellos I, Zacharakis E, Kanellos D, Pramateftakis MG, Tsachalis T, Betsis D. Long-term results after stapled haemorrhoidopexy for third-degree haemorrhoids. *Tech. Coloproctol.* 2006; 10: 47-49.

[18] Ravo B, Amato A, Bianco V, Bocassanta P, Bottini C, Carriero A, Milito G, Dodi G, Mascagni D, Orsini S, Pietroletti R, Ripetti V, Tagariello GB. Complications after stapled haemorrhoidectomy: can they be prevented? *Tech. Coloproctol.* 2002; 6: 83-88.

[19] Knight JS, Senapati A, Lamparelli MJ. National UK audit of procedure for prolapsing haemorrhoids on behalf of the Association of Coloproctology of Great Britain and Ireland. *Colorectal Dis.* 2008; 10: 440-445.

[20] Cheetham MJ, Cohen CRG, Kamm MA, Phillips RKS. A randomized controlled trial of diathermy hemorrhoidectomy vs stapled hemorrhoidectomy in an intended day-care setting with long-term follow-up. *Dis. Col. Rectum* 2003; 46: 491-497.

[21] Sutherland LM, Burchard AK, Matsuda K, Sweeney JL, Bokey EL, Childs PA, Roberts AK, Waxman BP, Maddern GJ. A systematic review of stapled haemorrhoidectomy. *Arch. Surg*. 2002; 137: 1395-1406.

[22] Wilson MS, Pope V, Doran HF, Fearn SJ, Brough WA. Objective comparison of stapled anopexy and open haemorrhoidectomy. *Dis. Col. Rectum* 2002; 45: 1437-1444.

[23] Herold A, Kirsch JI. Pain after stapled haemorrhoidopexy. *Lancet* 2000; 356: 2187.

[24] Maw A, Eu KW, Scow-Cohen F. Retroperitoneal sepsis complicating stapled hemorrhoidectomy. Report of a case and review of the literature. *Dis. Col. Rectum*. 2002; 45: 826-828.

In: Hemorrhoids: Symptoms, Diagnosis… ISBN: 978-1-60876-478-5
Authors: P. Salinitri et al., pp. 107-120

Chapter 5

EXCISION HEMORRHOIDECTOMY – NEW METHODS TO IMPROVE OUTCOMES OF AN OLD TECHNIQUE

***Kok-Yang Tan*[1] *and Francis Seow-Choen*[#]**
Department of Surgery, Alexandra Hospital, Singapore
#Seow-Choen Colorectal Centre, Singapore

ABSTRACT

Introduction

The lower cost of the procedure associated with a good long term cosmetic effect in patients with large skin tags make open excision hemorrhoidectomy a viable option still.

It is not uncommon however for surgical excision of hemorrhoids to be associated with postoperative pain together with perianal discharge, itchiness and irritation during the healing phase. Some recent local studies have provided us some insight into improving wound healing rates and postoperative pain after excision hemorrhoidectomy. This article reviews and discusses recent innovations of post-hemorrhoidectomy pain control and wound healing.

---

1 Correspondance: Kok-Yang TAN, Consultant Surgeon, Department of Surgery, Alexandra Hospital, 378 Alexandra Road, Singapore 159964, E-mail: kokyangtan@gmail.com.

Improving Outcome after Excision Hemorrhoidectomy

There is no doubt that postoperative spasm of the internal sphincter contributes to pain and poor wound healing. Topical glyceryl trinitrate (GTN) reduces anal canal pressures and improves anodermal blood flow. Post-hemorrhoidectomy topical use of GTN may reduce anal spasm and improve postoperative pain while improved anodermal blood flow may accelerate wound healing.

In another local study looking at the addition of methylene blue to local analgesics to prolong postoperative local anesthetic effect, we found that methylene blue was effective in prolonging anesthesia for up to about 3 weeks.

More recently, several randomized trials comparing diathermy haemorrhoidectomy to Ligasure hemorrhoidectomy have also found improvement in pain and healing using Ligasure. Dissection with Ligasure is associated with a reduced collateral damage to adjacent tissue compared to diathermy. The reduced anal spasm and smaller open wounds associated with Ligasure hemorrhoidectomy may have contributed to earlier wound healing.

Conclusion

Recent studies have provided some new methods for improving the postoperative outcomes of the technique of excision hemorrhoidectomy. Wound healing rates may be improved by topical glyceryl trinitrate which improves anodermal blood flow and also with the usage of Ligasure. The addition of methylene blue for topical analgesics may allow a prolongation of analgesic which may allow for a more painless recovery. More studies are currently being conducted for further improvement of results in an operation that is frequently indicated in our population.

INTRODUCTION

Although there is currently no doubt about the advantages of stapled hemorrhoidopexy,[1, 2] conventional open excision hemorrhoidectomy remains a frequently performed operation. The lower cost of the procedure associated with a good long term cosmetic effect in patients with large skin tags make open hemorrhoidectomy a viable option still. An Italian study published very recently actually found the Milligan-Morgan procedure to have better long-term results compared to stapled hemorrhoidopexy.[3] These results were echoed in a systematic review a few months prior.[4] In that review, 12 randomized trials comparing conventional excision hemorrhoidectomy to stapled hemorrhoidopexy were included. Follow-up periods ranged from 6 to 39 months with medians 7 – 14 months). Conventional hemorrhoidectomy was found to be more effective in preventing long-term recurrence of hemorrhoids (odds ratio (OR), 3.85; 95 percent CI 1.47–10.07; $P < 0.006$).

Furthermore one should be aware that at every level of prolapse, the hemorrhoidal tissues can be large or small.[1] Hence there are large circumferential 2nd degree hemorrhoids which may demand therapy because of incessant bleeding and small forth degree hemorrhoids where the main symptom is prolapsed and troublesome external components. While the former is optimally treated with stapled hemorrhoidopexy, excision hemorrhoidectomy may well produce better results in the latter.

It is not uncommon however, for surgical excision of hemorrhoids to be associated with postoperative pain together with perianal discharge, itchiness and irritation during the healing phase.[5] The amount of postoperative symptoms are highly variable, and depend on the severity of the hemorrhoidal disease, individual pain threshold, racial and cultural differences, quality and type of anesthesia, postoperative care, and the surgical technique. Some of these factors are more important than others in influencing post-operative pain and healing.[5]

Some recent studies have provided us some insight into improving wound healing rates and postoperative pain after excision hemorrhoidectomy.

Healing Process after Excision Hemorrhoidectomy

Immediately after the surgical trauma of hemorrhoidal excision, an acute local inflammatory response ensues. By day 6 after surgical excision, innate defense mechanisms and adaptive tissue response occurs where the wound develops an inflammatory cellular infiltration rich in macrophages and lymphoplasmacytic cells.[6] This response is likely responsible for the good wound healing of hemorrhoidectomy wounds despite abundant bacterial colonisation.[7]

There is no doubt that postoperative spasm of the internal sphincter contributes to pain and poor wound healing.[5, 8] Anal spasm may also further reduce the anodermal blood flow in a manner similar to that of chronic anal fissures and in doing so impair local adaptive tissue response and thus wound healing. The intensity of the anal spasm is to a certain extent affected by the surgical technique and it is likely to be aggravated by surgical injury of the internal anal sphincter.

In view of these factors discussed above, it makes sense that the optimal surgical excision involves minimal surgical trauma and inflicts the least amount of pain during the procedure and postoperative anal spasm should be addressed as much as possible.

OPTIMAL SURGICAL TECHNIQUE

In our standard conventional technique of excision hemorrhoidectomy, patients are placed in the lithotomy position and can be operated under general, regional or even local anaesthesia.[5] The perianal region and intersphincteric grooves are infiltrated with local anesthetic prior to dissection. Diathermy is used to dissect the hemorrhoidal tissue off the internal sphincter and the pedicle is secured using diathermy coagulation.[5] We have found it important to infiltrate the tissue locally adequately so as to reduce the pain during the procedure which will lead to reduced postoperative anal spasm and pain.

We compared the results between using scissors and diathermy for open hemorrhoidectomy.[9] Forty-nine consecutive patients with symptomatic prolapsed piles refractory to conservative treatment were randomized prospectively for conventional scissors excision with ligation or for diathermy excision.

There was a significantly shorter median time of surgery for the diathermy group ($p<0.05$). There was no statistically significant difference in the severity of postoperative pain between the two groups. However, the use of oral analgesics was significantly lower in the diathermy group ($p<0.02$).

After a median follow-up of 35 weeks in both groups, 3 patients in the scissors group and 1 patient in the diathermy group developed mild anal stricture, which were adequately treated by bulk laxatives alone. All wounds in both groups healed completely. There was no incidence of post-hemorrhoidectomy bleeding or anal incontinence in either group.

We concluded that diathermy excision of hemorrhoids was significantly faster than scissors excision, there was no need for ligation of the vascular pedicles, and there was a significant reduction in the oral analgesic requirements. The diathermy method does not cause any increase in early or late postoperative complications.

Another similar study of 135 patients also found that open haemorrhoidectomy was associated with less postoperative pain and patients in the diathermy group used less analgesic. There also was no increased risk of post-operative hemorrhage in the group without pedicle ligation.[10]

The use of diathermy is more advantageous over scissors as hemostasis is good and thus visibility of the internal sphincter is superior with reduced injury to the sphincter. Painful anal canal packing is also not required as a result of the superior hemostasis.

Parks first postulated that post-hemorrhoidectomy pain might be due to exposed and denuded anal sphincter resulting in anal spasm.[11] He thus advocated closing the hemorrhoidectomy wound.

We also conducted a study between closed and open hemorrhoidectomy using diathermy in a prospective randomized trial.[12] Open hemorrhoidectomy was performed without ligation of the pedicle, while in closed hemorrhoidectomy, the pedicle was transfixed and the mucosal wound edges were sutured with absorbable sutures.

Thirty-three patients underwent closed hemorrhoidectomy using diathermy and 34 patients underwent open hemorrhoidectomy using diathermy. There were also no differences in the postoperative pain score or analgesic requirement between the two groups. Although primary repair should lead to earlier wound healing and less pain in the closed hemorrhoidectomy group, this was not realized because of wound infection and dehiscence in 8 patients after closed hemorrhoidectomy.

A more recent meta-analysis of randomized controlled trials comparing open and close hemorrhoidectomy also did not find significant difference in postoperative pain.[13]

Surgical Excision Using Ligasure Vessel Sealing Device

Recently, we conducted a randomized trial comparing diathermy hemorrhoidectomy to Ligasure hemorrhoidectomy.14 We randomized 44 patients, 22 to Ligasure and 22 to diathermy. 43 patients were analyzed. They were aged between 19 and 71 years.

A standardized general anaesthetic technique using propofol, fentanyl and inhalation anaesthesia was used. All patients were given an enema prior to surgery. Patients underwent Milligan-Morgan open hemorrhoidectomy using either Ligasure or diathermy according to randomization. Injection of 10 mls of 0.25% bupivacaine into the perianal skin was performed prior to dissection in all cases. The pile masses were retracted and dissection was performed using either diathermy or Ligasure Vessel Sealing device off the internal sphincter. (Figure 1)

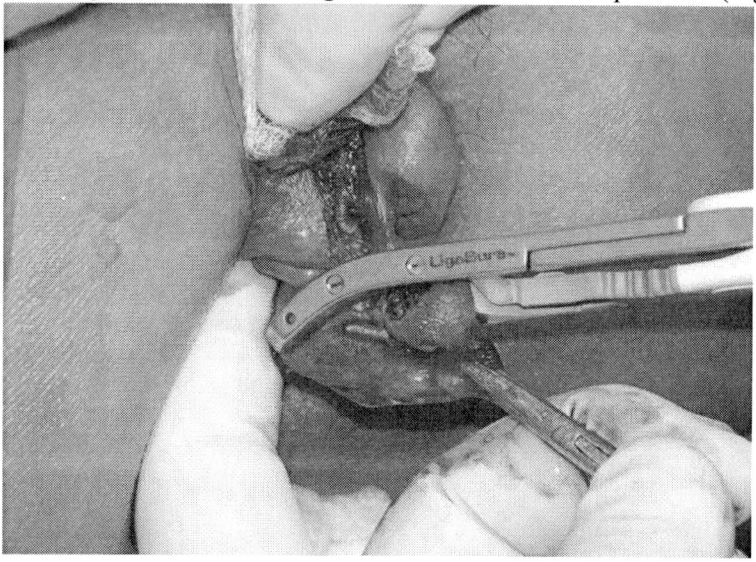

Figure 1. Dissection of the pile mass off the internal sphincter using the Ligasure Vessel Sealing Device

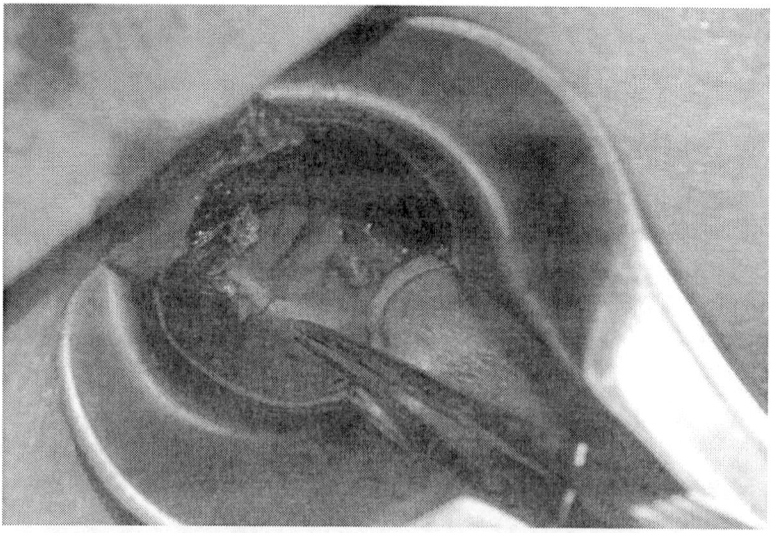

Figure 2. The pile mass has been excised. Coagulation with the Ligasure Vessel Sealing device leaves a line of coagulated tissue where the edges are relatively closely applied to each other. The pedicle is secured with the Ligasure device.

The pedicles were secured clear of the internal sphincter and the resected wound left open to granulate with adequate skin bridges. (Figure 2) Operative time was recorded by operating theater nurses. Blood lost was measured as the number of soaked gauzes.

Patients were acquainted with an 11 point visual analog pain score from 0 to 10. At home patients were asked to record their maximum pain score for the day before retiring. The patients also recorded the total number of analgesic tablets taken for that day. The patients' wounds were assessed at scheduled appointments. Wound healing was defined as complete epithelialization as seen on physical examination. The state of the wound was graded into 5 grades from sloughy to completely healed. A single assessor performed the assessment.

There were no differences in patient demographics and type of hemorrhoid being operated on. Ligasure hemorrhoidectomy had a significantly lower mean operative time and intraoperative bleeding. There was no statistically significant difference in the incidence of complications between the 2 groups. In this study, there was also no difference in postoperative pain of patients in both arms of the study. Sixty percent of patients who underwent Ligasure haemorrhoidectomy had wounds that were completely epithelized compared to 19% in the diathermy group at 3 weeks after surgery. At 3 weeks post surgery, hemorrhoidectomy performed with Ligasure had an odds ratio for complete epithelization of 3.1 over diathermy (95% CI 1.2 – 8.2).

Dissection with Ligasure is associated with a reduced collateral damage to adjacent tissue compared to diathermy. The reduced anal spasm and smaller open wounds associated with Ligasure hemorrhoidectomy may have contributed to earlier wound healing.

Subsequently, Nienhuijs and de Hingh performed a meta-analysis of 12 randomized trials comparing Ligasure to conventional hemorrhoidectomy including our trial that was described above.[15] A total of 1142 patients were included in the analysis. The pain score at the first day following surgery was significantly less in the Ligasure group when 835 patients from 10 studies were analysed. (Weighted Mean Differences (WMD) -2.07 CI -2.77 to -1.38). Most outcomes concerning analgesics used (7 studies) and pain scores up to 7 days (5 studies) favoured the Ligasure technique. There were no differences in complication rate between the Ligasure group and the conventional hemorrhoidectomy group.

From these findings, it can be concluded that Ligasure hemorrhoidectomy is superior in terms of postoperative pain and wound healing compared to conventional hemorrhoidectomy with no increase in postoperative complications. The disadvantage of the Ligasure technique however is the increased cost due to the disposable electrode.

ADJUNCTIVE MEASURES TO IMPROVE POSTOPERATIVE RESULTS

As discussed above postoperative spasm of the internal sphincter contributes to pain and poor wound healing. As such there had been many modifications of surgical technique to decrease this spasm in attempts to reduce pain and improve wound healing. Anal dilatation was used to reduce post-hemorrhoidectomy pain. However, this was associated with an increased risk of severe irreversible sphincter damage and anal incontinence. Hot perineal baths which is so frequently prescribed actually do not result in anal sphincter relaxation.[16]Another study found warm perineal baths to be not useful in reducing post-hemorrhoidectomy pain and wound healing.[17] We do not prescribe warm baths to our patients.

We investigated the use of internal anal sphincterotomy in conjunction with hemorrhoidectomy to reduce postoperative anal spasm.[18] Sixteen patients were randomized to hemorrhoidectomy only and 17 to hemorrhoidectomy and lateral sphincterotomy. There was no difference in postoperative pain scores and 2 patients in the sphincterotomy group continued to experienced distressing incontinence to liquid feces, symptoms persisting in 1 patient even after 1 year post surgery. Although there have been subsequent advocates of sphincterotomy during hemorrhoidectomy,[19, 20] we caution that the risk of such a procedure outweigh the potential benefits. The risk of incontinence after sphincterotomy is real[21] and this is especially so when it is used in hemorrhoidectomy where the potential to injure the internal sphincter is already increased. Potential improved postoperative pain is thus not justified when long-term risk of incontinence is possible.

The use of measures that only have a temporary effect thus is much more attractive. We studied the effect of trimebutine suppository (Proctolog) on post-hemorrhoidectomy pain.[22] Eighty patients were randomized to receive an application of Proctolog immediately after the procedure and another 80 did not receive a suppository in this randomized controlled study. An independent, blinded observer determined the pain scores. Although Proctolog reduced the resting anal pressure ($P < 0.001$), there were no differences in the pain score at 4 h after haemorrhoidectomy, maximum pain during the first 24 hours, maximum pain during the second postoperative day, ketoprofen requirement or need for intramuscular pethidine injections between the groups.

Topical glyceryl trinitrate (GTN) reduces anal canal pressures and improves anodermal blood flow.[23] Post-hemorrhoidectomy topical use of GTN may reduce anal spasm and improve postoperative pain while improved anodermal blood flow may accelerate wound healing.

A randomized, prospective, double-blind placebo-controlled trial on 82 patients undergoing diathermy hemorrhoidectomy was conducted.[24] Patients were randomized to either 0.2% GTN ointment (RectogesicTM—Cellegy Australia Pty Ltd, 203 New South Head Road, Edgecliff NSW 2027, Australia) or placebo (vaseline) ointment applied topically to the perianal region after open diathermy hemorrhoidectomy.

There were 40 patients in the GTN ointment arm and 42 patients in the placebo arm. There were no statistically significant differences in the sex, weight, type of hemorrhoid, type of surgery (emergency or elective), number of hemorrhoids excised, duration of surgery, hospital stay and complication rate. By week 3 however, 17 of patients in the GTN arm had completely epithelized wounds compared to 8 of patients in the placebo arm. (p=0.021). Only 1 patient in the GTN arm experienced headaches requiring discontinuation of the ointment.

We concluded that glyceryl trinitrate (0.2%) ointment is useful in improving the wound healing rates. However, there was no significant effect on postoperative pain.

Other studies using adjunctive pharmacology to reduce post-hemorrhoidectomy anal spasm are summarized in Table 1.[25-30] It can be seen that the effect on postoperative pain is not consistent and no clear conclusion can be drawn from available studies on their efficacy at the moment. It is likely that other factors including inflammation and bacterial colonization, affect postoperative pain as well.

On the other hand, the effect of these adjunctive measures on wound healing seems to be more consistent. This is clinically significant as patients will suffer from reduced perianal irritation and discharge and have an earlier return to normal activity.

The effect of trying to reduce infection of the post-hemorrhoidectomy wound has been studied.[31, 32] Oral metronidazole was compared to placebo in the randomized trials. Both studies found reduced secondary pain and earlier return to work.

Another useful adjunct is micronized flavonidic fraction. A randomized trial was conducted on 228 patients.[33] Patients were randomized to micronized flavonidic fraction for a period of 1 week or placebo.

Table 1. Pharmacological Methods to Reduce Postoperative Anal Spasm

Study	Agent	Pain Scores	Analgesic use	Wound Healing
Ho et al[22] 1997 Randomized	Trimebutine suppository	Not significantly reduced		Not studied
Wasvary et al [25] 2001 Randomized	GTN ointment 0.2%	Not significantly reduced	Significantly less only on day 2	Not studied
Hwang et al[26] 2003 Randomized	GTN ointment 0.2%	Significantly reduced	Not significantly reduced	Significantly improved
Tan et al[24] 2006 Randomized	GTN ointment 0.2%	Not significantly reduced	Not significantly reduced	Significantly improved
Silverman et al[27] 2005 Randomized	Calcium channel blocker ointment	Significantly reduced	Not significantly reduced	Not studied
Davies et al[29] 2003 Randomized	Botulinum toxin injection	Significantly reduced day 6 and 7	Not significantly reduced	Not studied
Patti et al[28] 2005	Botulinum toxin injection	Not studied	Not studied	Significantly improved
Singh et al[30] 2009	Botulinum toxin injection	Not significantly reduced	Not studied	Not studied

While there was no difference in postoperative analgesic use, the risk of secondary bleeding was significantly reduced.

From the results of these studies, it can be inferred that the symptom of post-hemorrhoidectomy pain is indeed multifactorial and there is no single magic bullet that will improve pain consistently. The key to achieving good postoperative pain is a combination of good surgical technique and adequate adjunctive measures.

Recent Innovations

More recently, we have found the addition of methylene blue to local analgesics to prolong post-operative local anesthetic effect was effective in prolonging anesthesia for up to about 3 weeks.[34] Methylene blue has been widely used as a biological dye. We have found anecdotally that patients with perianal fistulae in whom we used methylene blue to delineate the tracts had less postoperative pain. A review of the literature revealed that intradermal injection methylene blue has been used successfully in intractable pruritus ani.[35] The mechanism of action of methylene blue is likely the destruction of dermal nerve endings.[35] Eusebio et al [36] were unable to demonstrate cutaneous nerve endings on electron microscopy in perianal skin punch biopsies after methylene blue therapy. We are currently investigating the use of methylene blue in addition to local anesthesia for patients undergoing excision hemorrhoidectomy.

Conclusion

Recent local studies have provided some new methods for improving the postoperative outcomes of the technique of excision hemorrhoidectomy. Wound healing rates may be improved by topical glyceryl trinitrate which improves anodermal blood flow and also with the usage of Ligasure. The addition of methylene blue for topical analgesics may allow a prolongation of analgesic which may allow for a more painless recovery. More studies are currently being conducted for further improvement of results in an operation that is frequently indicated in our population.

References

[1] Seow-Choen F, Tan KY. Hemorrhoids. *In* Bland KI, Büchler MW, Csendes A, et al., eds. General Surgery: Principles and International Practice 3rd Edition: *Springer*, 2009. pp. 857-864.

[2] Seow-Choen F. Stapled haemorrhoidectomy: pain or gain. *Br. J. Surg.* 2001; 88(1):1-3.

[3] Mattana C, Coco C, Manno A, et al. Stapled hemorrhoidopexy and Milligan Morgan hemorrhoidectomy in the cure of fourth-degree hemorrhoids: long-

term evaluation and clinical results. Dis Colon Rectum 2007; 50(11):1770-5.
[4] Jayaraman S, Colquhoun PH, Malthaner RA. Stapled hemorrhoidopexy is associated with a higher long-term recurrence rate of internal hemorrhoids compared with conventional excisional hemorrhoid surgery. *Dis. Colon. Rectum*. 2007; 50(9):1297-305.
[5] Tan KY, Seow-Choen F. The Operative Treatment by, and Results of, Diathermy Haemorrhoidectomy *In* Khubchandani IT, Paonessa N, Azimuddin K, eds. Surgical Treatment of Hemorrhoids 2nd Edition. London: Springer-Verlag, 2009. pp. 105-112.
[6] de Paula PR, Matos D, Franco M, et al. Why do anal wounds heal adequately? A study of the local immunoinflammatory defense mechanisms. *Dis. Colon. Rectum.* 2004; 47(11):1861-7.
[7] de Paula PR, Speranzini MB, Hamzagic HC, et al. Bacteriology of the anal wound after open hemorrhoidectomy. Qualitative and quantitative analysis. *Dis. Colon. Rectum.* 1991; 34(8):664-9.
[8] Cheetham MJ, Phillips RK. Evidence-based practice in haemorrhoidectomy. *Colorectal Dis*. 2001; 3(2):126-34.
[9] Seow-Choen F, Ho YH, Ang HG, Goh HS. Prospective, randomized trial comparing pain and clinical function after conventional scissors excision/ligation vs. diathermy excision without ligation for symptomatic prolapsed hemorrhoids. *Dis. Colon Rectum.* 1992; 35(12):1165-9.
[10] Bassi R, Bergami G. [The surgical treatment of hemorrhoids: diathermocoagulation and traditional technics. A prospective randomized study]. *Minerva Chir.* 1997; 52(4):387-91.
[11] Parks AG. The surgical treatment of haemorrhoids. *Br. J. Surg.* 1956; 43(180):337-51.
[12] Ho YH, Seow-Choen F, Tan M, Leong AF. Randomized controlled trial of open and closed haemorrhoidectomy. *Br. J. Surg.* 1997; 84(12):1729-30.
[13] Ho YH, Buettner PG. Open compared with closed haemorrhoidectomy: meta-analysis of randomized controlled trials. *Tech. Coloproctol.* 2007; 11(2):135-43.
[14] Tan KY, Zin T, Sim HL, et al. Randomized clinical trial comparing LigaSure haemorrhoidectomy with open diathermy haemorrhoidectomy. *Tech. Coloproctol.* 2008; 12(2):93-7.
[15] Nienhuijs S, de Hingh I. Conventional versus LigaSure hemorrhoidectomy for patients with symptomatic Hemorrhoids. *Cochrane Database Syst. Rev.* 2009(1):CD006761.

[16] Pinho M, Correa JC, Furtado A, Ramos JR. Do hot baths promote anal sphincter relaxation? *Dis. Colon Rectum.* 1993; 36(3):273-4.

[17] Gupta PJ. Warm sitz bath does not reduce symptoms in posthaemorrhoidectomy period: a randomized, controlled study. *ANZ. J. Surg.* 2008; 78(5):398-401.

[18] Mathai V, Ong BC, Ho YH. Randomized controlled trial of lateral internal sphincterotomy with haemorrhoidectomy. *Br. J. Surg.* 1996; 83(3):380-2.

[19] Galizia G, Lieto E, Castellano P, et al. Lateral internal sphincterotomy together with haemorrhoidectomy for treatment of haemorrhoids: a randomised prospective study. *Eur. J. Surg.* 2000; 166(3):223-8.

[20] Kanellos I, Zacharakis E, Christoforidis E, et al. Usefulness of lateral internal sphincterotomy in reducing postoperative pain after open hemorrhoidectomy. *World J. Surg.* 2005; 29(4):464-8.

[21] Ommer A, Wenger FA, Rolfs T, Walz MK. Continence disorders after anal surgery--a relevant problem? *Int. J. Colorectal Dis.* 2008; 23(11):1023-31.

[22] Ho YH, Seow-Choen F, Low JY, et al. Randomized controlled trial of trimebutine (anal sphincter relaxant) for pain after haemorrhoidectomy. *Br. J. Surg.* 1997; 84(3):377-9.

[23] Kua KB, Kocher HM, Kelkar A, Patel AG. Effect of topical glyceryl trinitrate on anodermal blood flow in patients with chronic anal fissures. *ANZ J. Surg.* 2001; 71(9):548-50.

[24] Tan KY, Sng KK, Tay KH, et al. Randomized clinical trial of 0.2 per cent glyceryl trinitrate ointment for wound healing and pain reduction after open diathermy haemorrhoidectomy. *Br. J. Surg.* 2006; 93(12):1464-8.

[25] Wasvary HJ, Hain J, Mosed-Vogel M, et al. Randomized, prospective, double-blind, placebo-controlled trial of effect of nitroglycerin ointment on pain after hemorrhoidectomy. *Dis. Colon. Rectum.* 2001; 44(8):1069-73.

[26] Hwang DY, Yoon SG, Kim HS, et al. Effect of 0.2 percent glyceryl trinitrate ointment on wound healing after a hemorrhoidectomy: results of a randomized, prospective, double-blind, placebo-controlled trial. *Dis. Colon. Rectum.* 2003; 46(7):950-4.

[27] Silverman R, Bendick PJ, Wasvary HJ. A randomized, prospective, double-blind, placebo-controlled trial of the effect of a calcium channel blocker ointment on pain after hemorrhoidectomy. *Dis. Colon. Rectum.* 2005; 48(10):1913-6.

[28] Patti R, Almasio PL, Muggeo VM, et al. Improvement of wound healing after hemorrhoidectomy: a double-blind, randomized study of botulinum toxin injection. *Dis. Colon. Rectum.* 2005; 48(12):2173-9.

[29] Davies J, Duffy D, Boyt N, et al. Botulinum toxin (botox) reduces pain after hemorrhoidectomy: results of a double-blind, randomized study. *Dis. Colon. Rectum*. 2003; 46(8):1097-102.

[30] Singh B, Box B, Lindsey I, et al. Botulinum toxin reduces anal spasm but has no effect on pain after haemorrhoidectomy. *Colorectal. Dis.* 2009; 11(2):203-7.

[31] Carapeti EA, Kamm MA, McDonald PJ, Phillips RK. Double-blind randomised controlled trial of effect of metronidazole on pain after day-case haemorrhoidectomy. *Lancet* 1998; 351(9097):169-72.

[32] Al-Mulhim AS, Ali AM, Al-Masuod N, Alwahidi A. Post hemorrhoidectomy pain. A randomized controlled trial. *Saudi Med. J.* 2006; 27(10):1538-41.

[33] Ho YH, Foo CL, Seow-Choen F, Goh HS. Prospective randomized controlled trial of a micronized flavonidic fraction to reduce bleeding after haemorrhoidectomy. *Br. J. Surg.* 1995; 82(8):1034-5.

[34] Tan KY, Seow-Choen F. Methylene blue injection reduces pain after lateral anal sphincterotomy. *Tech. Coloproctol.* 2007; 11(1):68-9.

[35] Farouk R, Lee PW. Intradermal methylene blue injection for the treatment of intractable idiopathic pruritus ani. *Br .J. Surg.* 1997; 84(5):670.

[36] Eusebio EB, Graham J, Mody N. Treatment of intractable pruritus ani. *Dis. Colon. Rectum*. 1990; 33(9):770-2.

In: Hemorrhoids: Symptoms, Diagnosis... ISBN: 978-1-60876-478-5
Authors: P. Salinitri et al., pp. 121-147

Chapter 6

VIDEOANOSCOPE ASSISTED STAPLED HEMORRHOIDOPEXY: A NOVEL PROCEDURE

Ali Dogan Bozdag[1]
Third Surgical Clinic of Izmir Ataturk Training and Research Hospital, Izmir – Turkey

ABSTRACT

Stapled hemorrhoidopexy is increasingly practiced in treatment of hemorrhoidal disease. For an ideal application of this method, purse-string suture must be put at a certain distance with appropriate thickness. This may sometimes be difficult, and an unsuitable purse string suture placement may increase the risk of postoperative complications. The videoanoscope was created to prevent the difficulties during application of the purse-string suture.

The videoanoscope consists of three pieces: the front piece with an open top gradually narrows and makes a nozzle at the tip; the top piece is a sliding lid that covers the front piece; and the back piece has a handle that allows insertion of a 10 mm telescope in order to shed light inside the anoscope and transfer images to the monitor.

The sliding lid forms a window above the anoscope when pulled back, and allows suturing rectal mucosa that hangs down into the anoscope.

1 Corresponding Author: Associate Professor Dr. Ali Dogan BOZDAG Mithatpasa Caddesi 388/7 35280 Asansor, Izmir – TURKEY Phone: +90 232 4252588, GSM: +90 532 4371597, Fax: +90 232 2434848, e-mail: bozdaga@gmail.com.

Suturing may be continued by rotating the anoscope clockwise direction, and it is completed upon reaching the start point.

The purse-string suture placement and the stapled haemorrhoidopexy procedure were easily performed by using the videoanoscope. Additionally, it is possible to get the view inside of the anoscope, and the procedure can be viewed on a monitor. Moreover it has some advantages such as recording the operation by videoanoscope, and these records may be useful for surgical training.

Introduction

Stapled hemorrhoidopexy, a method alternative to conventional hemorrhoidal surgery, is being more commonly performed nowadays for treatment of hemorrhoidal disease. Major facts why this method has become the reason for choice over the conventional method are less post-operative pain and earlier recovery [1]. In order to achieve the desired success using the stapled hemorrhoidopexy procedure, the purse string suture must cross at equal distances from linea dentata and must only include the mucosa and the submucosal layer; otherwise an ideal purse string suture cannot be referred to [2,3]. Various factors may lead to a non-ideal purse string suture. For example, internal hemorrhoids and loose rectal mucosa may prolapse to fill in the anoscope leading to a blocked vision and limited movements of the needle [2-7]. Several anoscope modifications have been reported in order to overcome such problems [2-5,8]. Similarly, we felt the need to modify the anoscope used in putting purse string suture a while after we had started performing stapled hemorrhoidopexy procedure at 2001 in our clinic [2,3]. We then developed the videoanoscope by the help of experience we gained using such modified anoscopes in order to put the purse string suture more reliably and to record the surgery [4]. The videoanoscope has been built using transparent acrylic material (Orthoacryl®, Dentaurum, Pforzheim, Germany) and can be sterilized by ethylene oxide before use. Patients are acknowledged before the procedure and signed informed consents are obtained.

Technical Specifications of the Videoanoscope:

1) The videoanoscope consists of three pieces (Figures 1 and 2).

2) The front piece is made up of an open-top conical-shaped cylinder that narrows at the tip. Secondly, a sliding lid can be placed on top of the front piece (Figures 3 and 4).
3) The sliding lid allows the surgeon to adjust the extent to which the anoscope's window is desired to be opened and the amount of mucosa entering the window.
4) The back piece consists of a hollow handle inside which a 10-mm, 0-degree telescope used in laparoscopic surgery can be placed. By this combination, the surgery area can be illuminated and the view can be transferred to the monitor (Figure 5).
5) The front and the back pieces are attached to each other by a lock mechanism which can be unlocked allowing the two pieces to be disconnected (Figures 6 and 7).

Surgical Technique:

1) The patient is prepared for surgery in Jackknife position following spinal anesthesia (Figures 8-10).
2) Needle of the 26 mm atraumatic polypropylene is inserted through the window inside the videoanoscope (Figures 11 and 12).
3) The videoanoscope is inserted into the rectum by applying a lubricant to its tip (Figures 13-15).
4) The telescope is placed inside the handle at the back of the videoanoscope providing light at the inside of the videoanoscope and eliminating the need to light sources such as surgery room lamps (Figures 16-18).
5) Sutures can be put on rectal mucosa which enters the adjustable window of the videoanoscope. Special attention is exerted to prevent any mucosal gap between each bite of the purse string suture. So that the polypropilene suture material is kept under tension to see the end point of the suture and the following suture is passed through the mucosa very close to the previous one. On reaching the starting point, a complete purse string suture is achieved by rotating the anoscope clockwise which allows the sutures to be put at equal distances from linea dentata (Figures 19-22).
6) Isotonic saline solution is injected submucosally before each mucosal suture is put (Figure 23).

7) All people in the surgery room can watch the procedure since the view is transferred to the monitor. The surgeon can put sutures by looking at either the anoscope or by watching the monitor (Figures 24 and 25).
8) On completion of the purse string suture, the back piece remains inside the rectum while the front piece containing a lid is removed (Figures 26 and 27).
9) A PPH03 (Ethicon-Endosurgery, Cincinnati, OH, USA) stapler is placed inside the rectum by passing through the back piece. The purse string suture is tightened and tied while the anvil is in (Figures 28 and 29).
10) Hemostasis is maintained after a 180-second wait time, the first 90 seconds of which is spent following closure of the stapler and the second 90 seconds following firing (Figure 30)
11) Stapler is removed and the ring is checked (Figure 31).
12) Same procedures can be applied using a 34-mm Stapler (34 mm, CEEA stapler; Tyco, Norwalk, CT) (Figures 32-35).
13) Stapler line is checked and, if necessary, hemostatic suture is put while the back piece of the videoanoscope is located inside anal canal (Figures 36 and 37).
14) The operation is concluded by placing a spongosten inside anal canal (Figures 38-40).

Conclusion

In principle, the purse string suture must cross at a constant distance, approximately 4 cm from linea dentata and be sustained continually by including the mucosa and the submucosal layer. Sustaining the suture continually is assured mainly by insertion of the needle right next to the point that it exits the mucosa [2,3]. Consequent sutures may not be applied the same way in case the suture area is blocked by large internal hemorrhoids or loose rectal mucosa that fills in the anoscope. Viewable area will be blocked and the needle's movements will be limited if a hemorrhage occurs from the mucosa or by penetration of the needle into the hemorrhoid [2,6,7]. As a result, at some locations, the purse string suture may cross closer to linea dentata, cross shallower or deeper tissues, or not cross at all leading to closer location of stapler line to linea dentata, occurrence of thinner or thicker sections, or missing parts of the ring, respectively [6,9-12]. Several problems may occur in such cases. For example, a stapled line closer to linea dentata may cause resistant pain and incontinence [10]; a ring with disrupted integrity or weaker sections may enhance bleeding risk or lead to recurrences in long term [13]; the resected ring may include deeper structures in the case of a deeper purse string suture which may lead to bleeding, hematoma and pelvic sepsis [14,15]. Various complications caused by difficulties in applying the technique or technical errors have been described in the literature [1-5,7-9]. We believe that principally the purse string suture is referred to by “the technique” since the purse string suture stage ultimately requires the surgeon’s talent during stapled hemorrhoidopexy procedure and the stapler only resects and staples the tissue collected inside the anvil regardless of how and where the purse string suture was placed [2,3]. The above-mentioned problems can be overcome by putting the purse string suture ideally. A previous study reported that placing the stapler line with a constant distance from linea dentata of 22 mm reduced the need for narcotic analgesics and caused the patients to return to work earlier [1].

Preventing the hemorrhoids to fill in the anoscope may help putting the purse string suture more conveniently. It has been reported that purse string suture is put more conveniently and almost ideally using modified anoscopes [2-5,8, 16]. We modified the purse string suture anoscope for several times in our clinic and, finally, invented the videoanoscope at 2006.

The videoanoscope has additional advantages over other modified anoscopes. First of all, the sliding lid of the videoanoscope prevents the prolapse of loose tissues to fill inside the anoscope and block the vision. The sliding lid is pulled open to a distance that is determined according to the amount of mucosa desired to enter the window by the surgeon [4]. In other words, the sliding lid helps the surgeon to determine and check the amount of mucosa to be sutured. It has been reported that submucosal injection of isotonic saline solution separates the rectal mucosa and submucosa layers from muscularis propria helping the surgeon to include only the mucosa and submucosa inside the resected ring [17]. Injection of isotonic saline solution into the half moon-shaped mucosa and putting sutures can be easily performed using the videoanoscope. The anoscope becomes half-open upon removal of the sliding lid allowing the surgeon to fully visualize the surgical area, check the purse string suture, and make interventions when needed. Videoanoscope also allows capturing a close-up of the surgical area and transferring the video to a monitor. Therefore, the operation field was extended for the surgeon by using the monitor during the procedure. The primary assistant doctor in the surgery team can assist the surgeon by watching the monitor rather than by trying to look inside the anoscope which limits the movements of the surgeon, and the surgeon can put the purse string suture by either looking at the surgical area or watching the monitor. The fact that all stages of the surgery can be visualized by not only the surgeon and the assistant doctor but also by all people in the surgery room serves advantages during both the purse string suture stage and the bleeding control stage of stapler line. In addition, the fact that the videoanoscope allows the surgery to be recorded may help to improve the education of general surgery [4]. In conclusion, "videoanoscope-assisted stapled hemorrhoidopexy" is a more controlled method that is suitable with general surgical principles and reliable due to its additional advantages over other anoscopes.

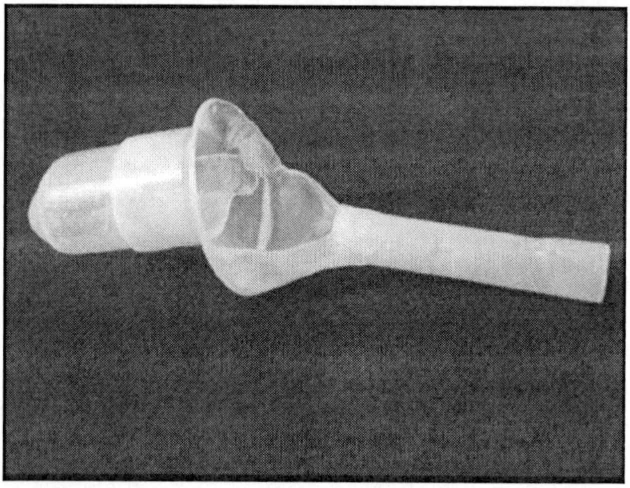

Figure 1.Videoanoscope

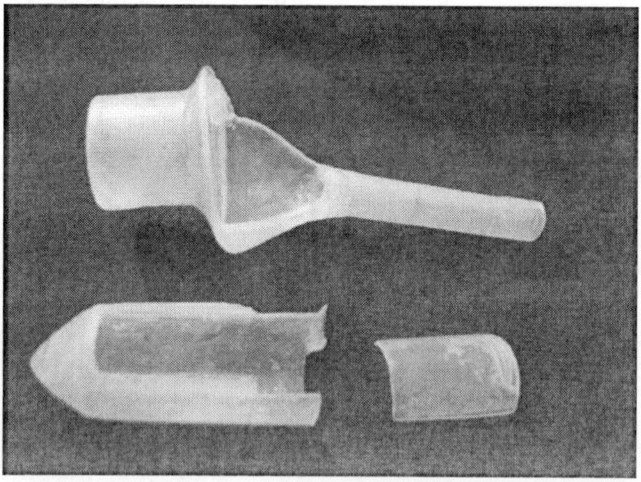

Figure 2.Videoanoscope consists of three pieces.

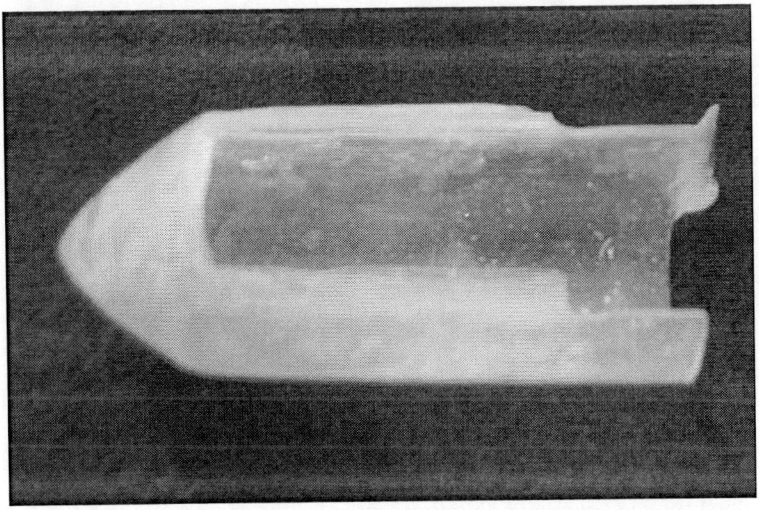

Figure 3.The front piece is made up of an open-top conical-shaped cylinder that narrows at the tip

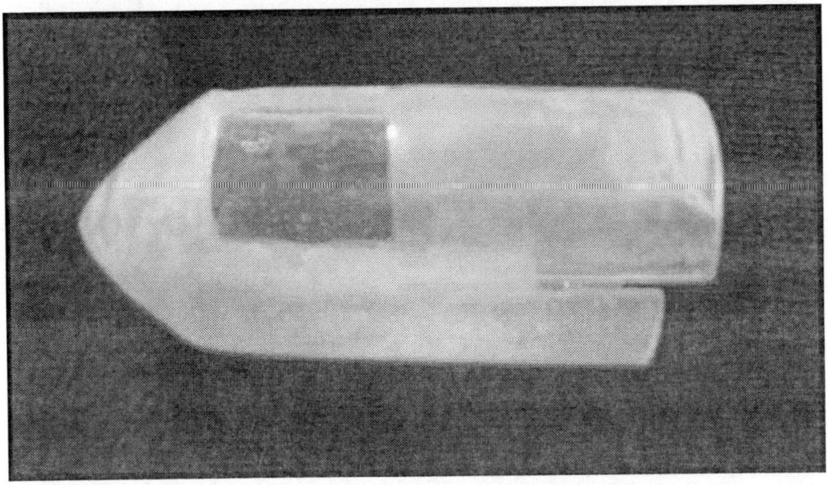

Figure 4.The second piece is a sliding lid used to open and close the top of the front piece.

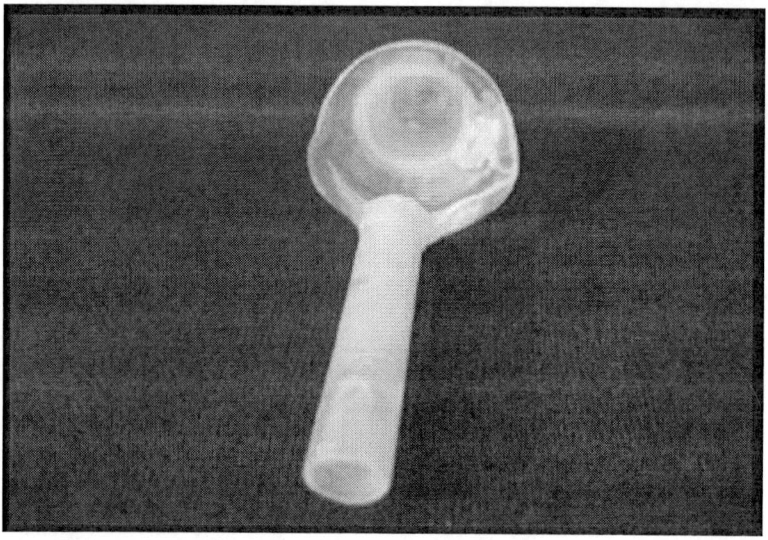

Figure 5. The back piece contains a hollow handle inside which a 10-mm telescope can be placed.

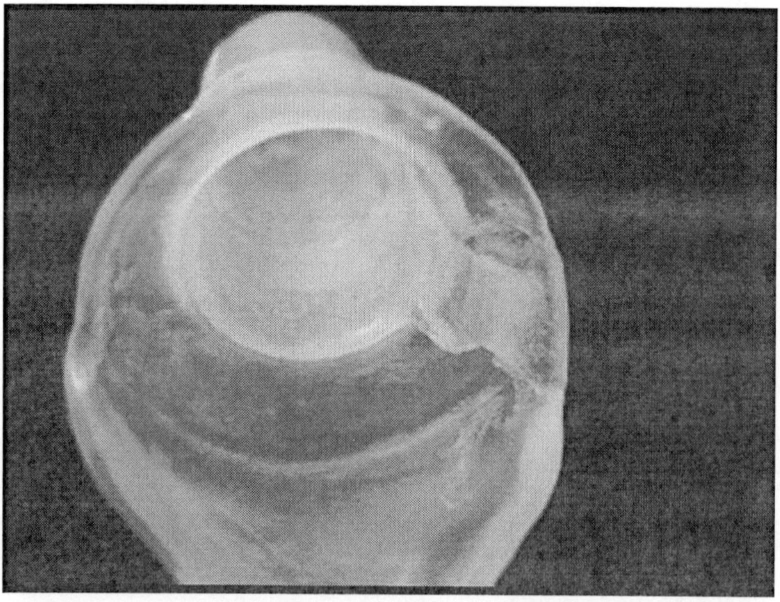

Figure 6.The front and the back pieces are locked to each other.

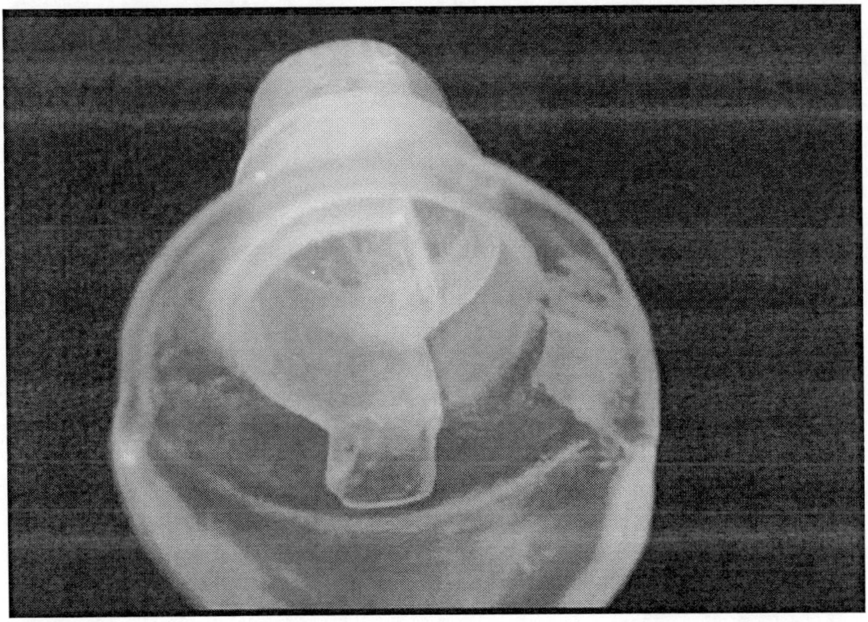

Figure 7.The front and back pieces are disassociated by rotating the front piece .

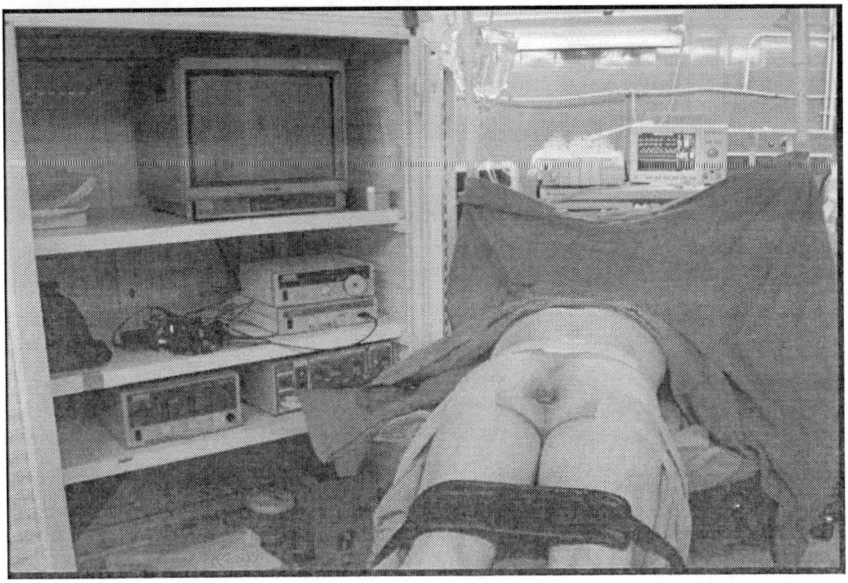

Figure 8.The patient is prepared for surgery in Jackknife position following spinal anesthesia .

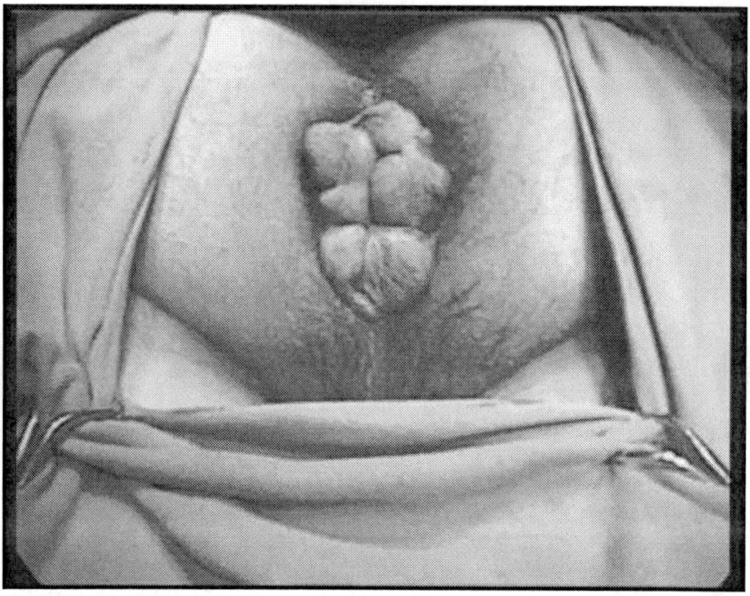

Figure 9. External hemorrhoids of the patient who has grade IV hemorrhoidal disease.

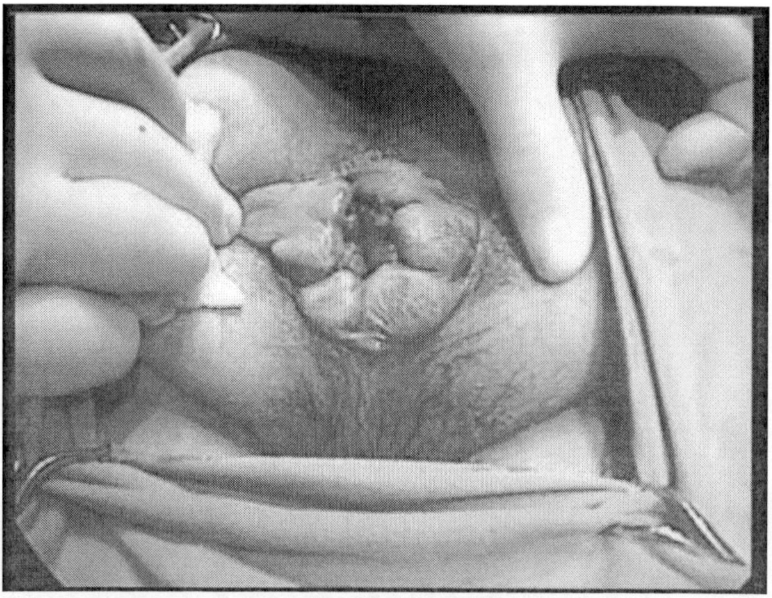

Figure 10. External and internal hemorrhoids of the patient who has grade IV hemorrhoidal disease .

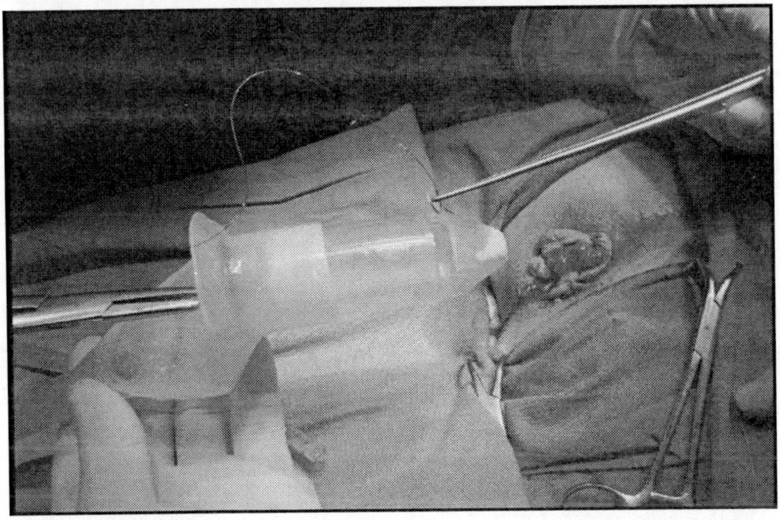

Figure 11.The needle of the 2/0 atraumatic propylene is inserted inside the videoanoscope by opening the sliding lid.

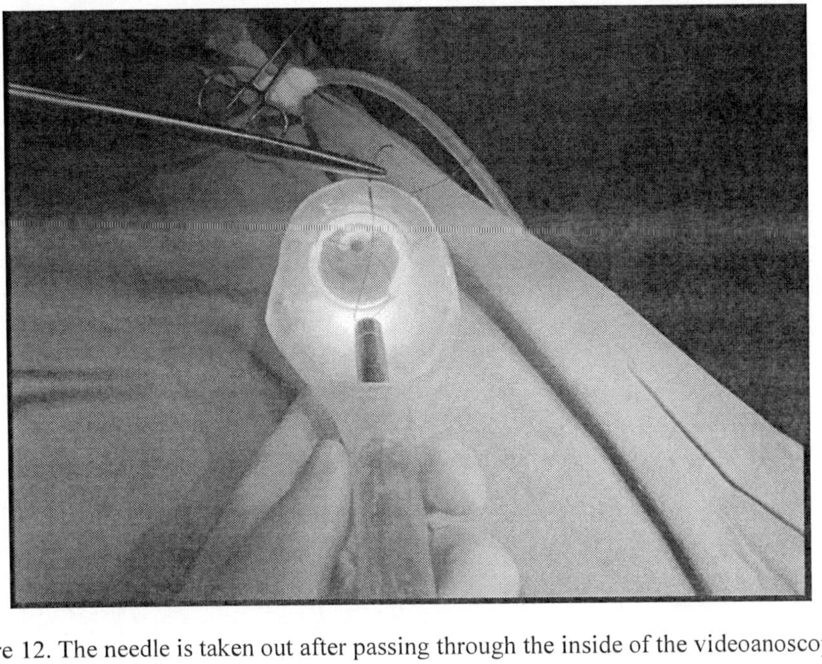

Figure 12. The needle is taken out after passing through the inside of the videoanoscope which is illuminated by the telescope .

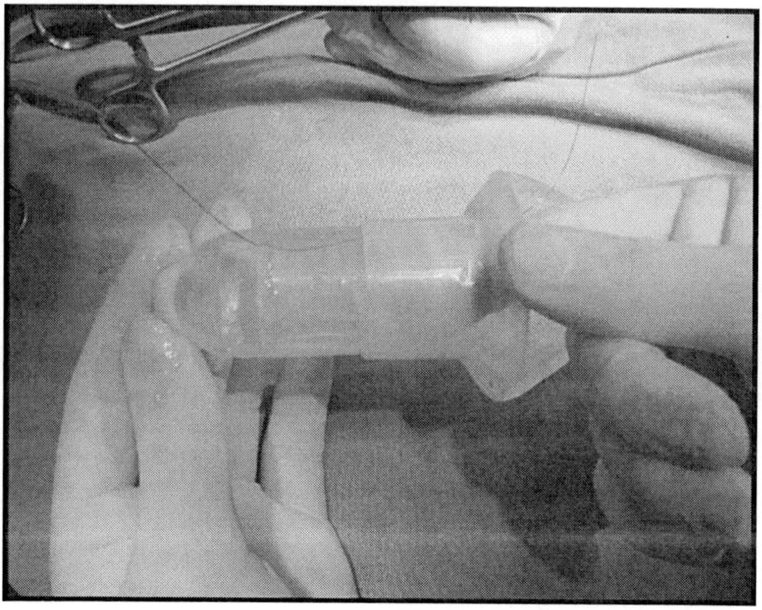

Figure 13. A lubricant is applied to the tip of the videoanoscope.

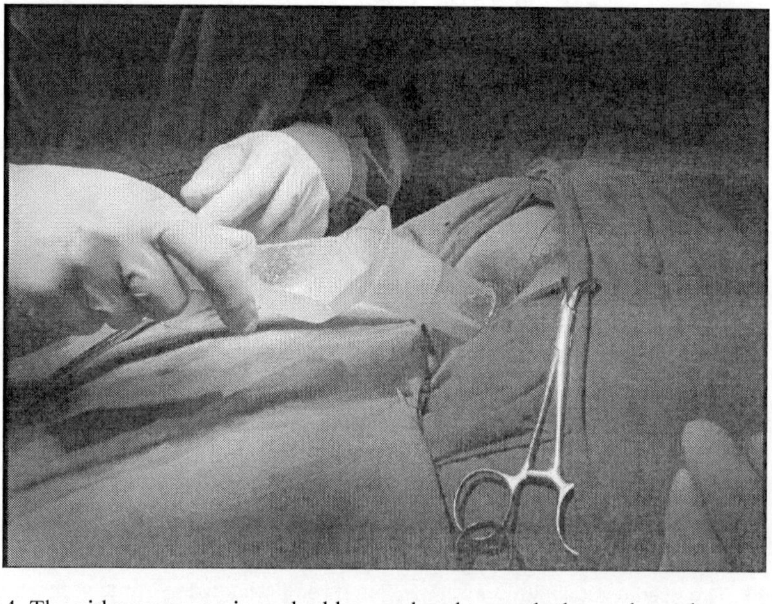

Figure 14. The videoanoscope is pushed by one hand towards the anal canal.

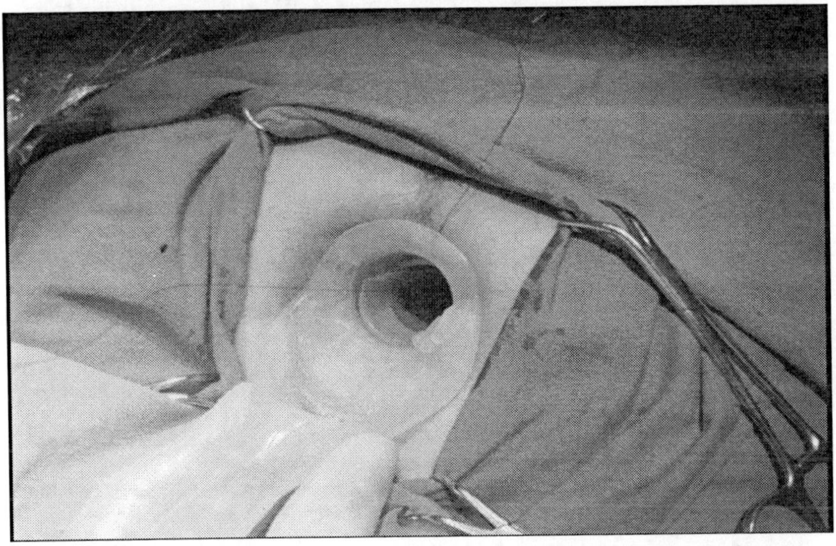

Figure 15. The videoanoscope is inserted inside the rectum easily due to its ergonomic structure.

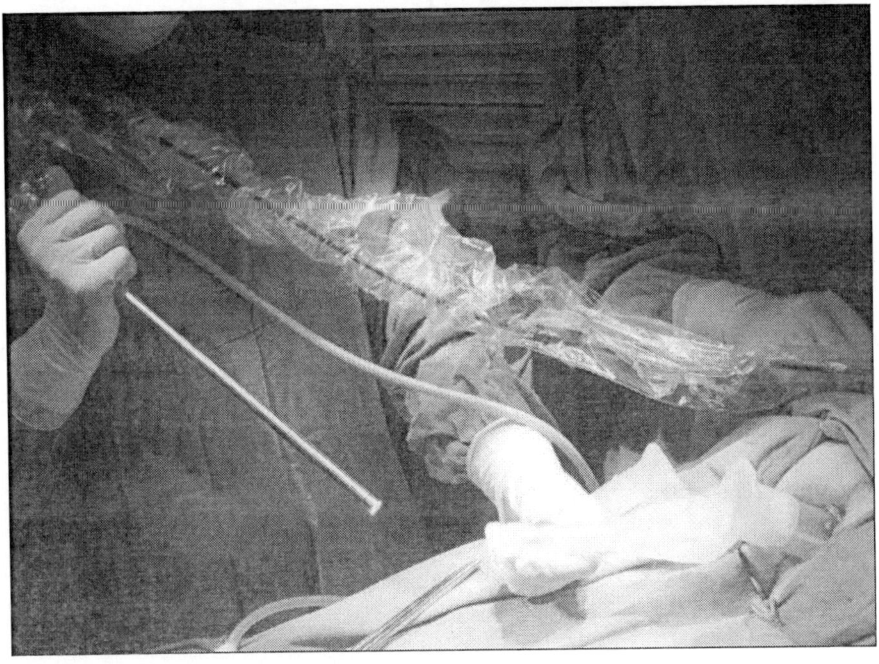

Figure 16.The telescope is directed towards the back piece.

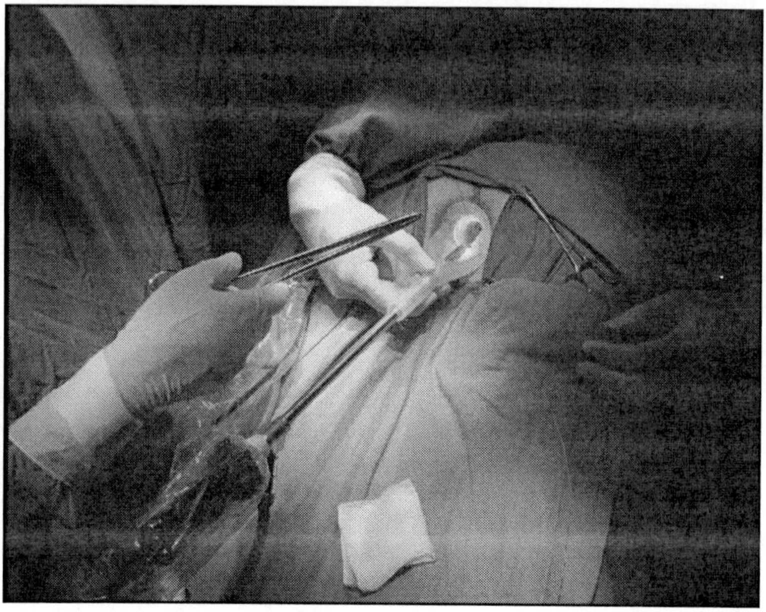

Figure 17.The surgeon is prepared for putting sutures .

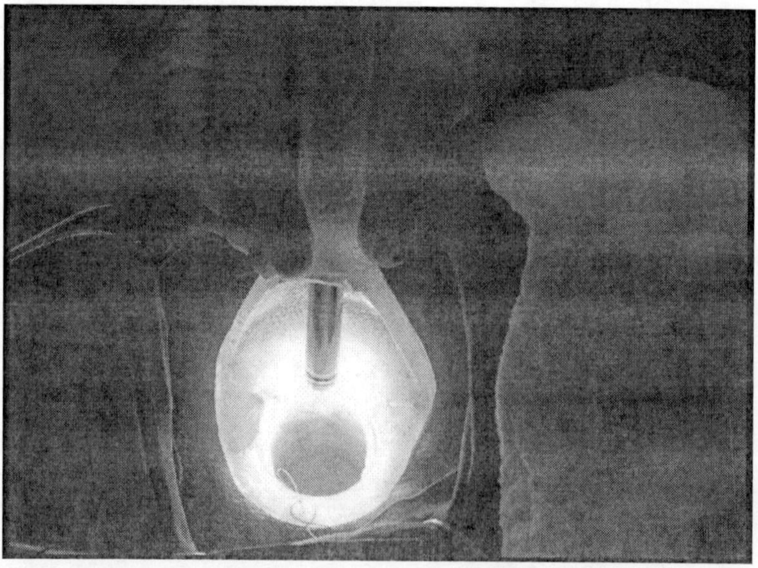

Figure 18.The telescope illuminates the inside of the videoanoscope .

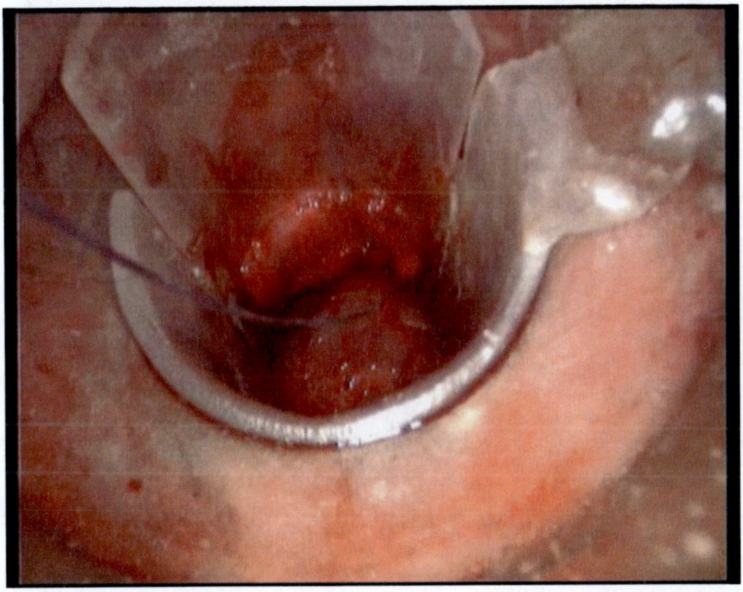

Figure 19. **The sliding lid allows the surgeon to adjust the extent to which the anoscope's** window is desired to be opened and the amount of mucosa entering the window.

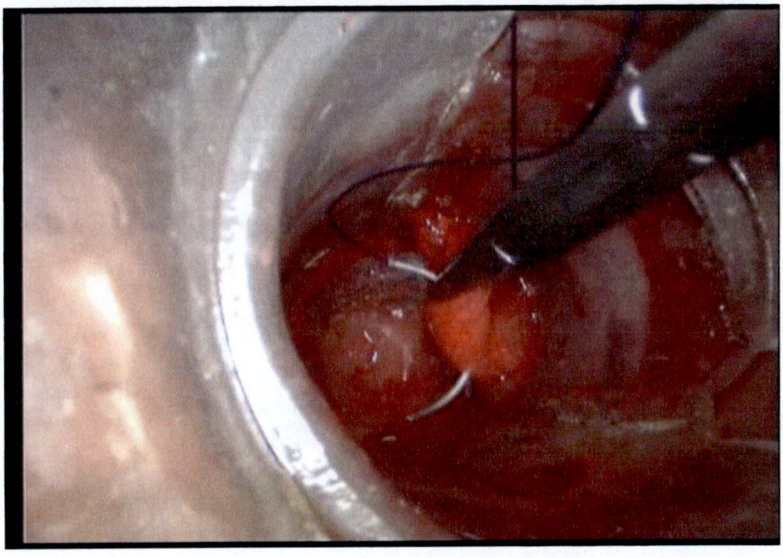

Figure 20. Sutures are put through the rectum mucosa entering the window.

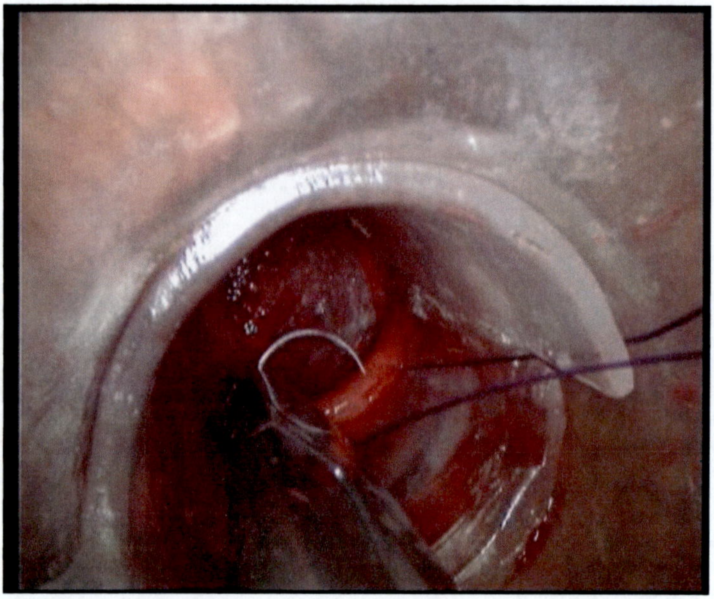

Figure 21.Suturing is continued by rotating the videoanoscope clockwise.

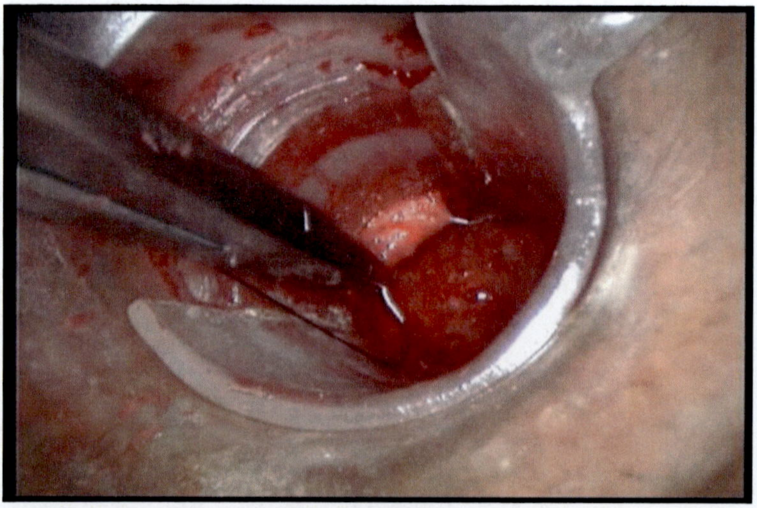

Figure 22. The purse string suture is put at equal distances and completed by reaching the starting point .

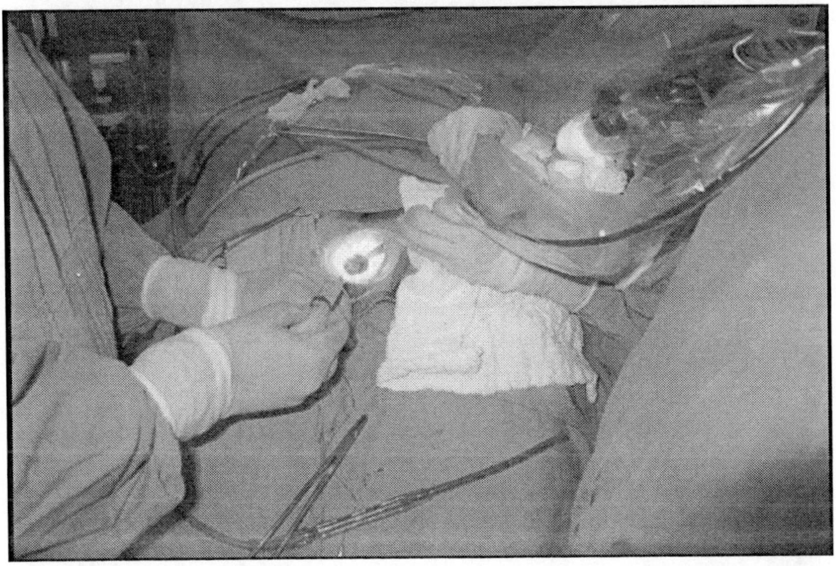

Figure 23. Physiological serum is injected submucosally before each suture is put.

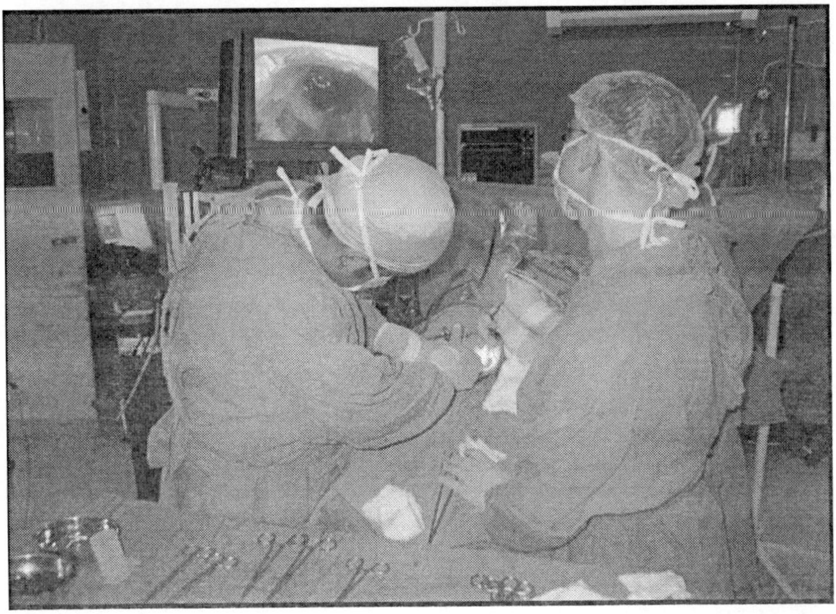

Figure 24. The view of the surgical area is transferred to the monitor during the procedure of putting sutures.

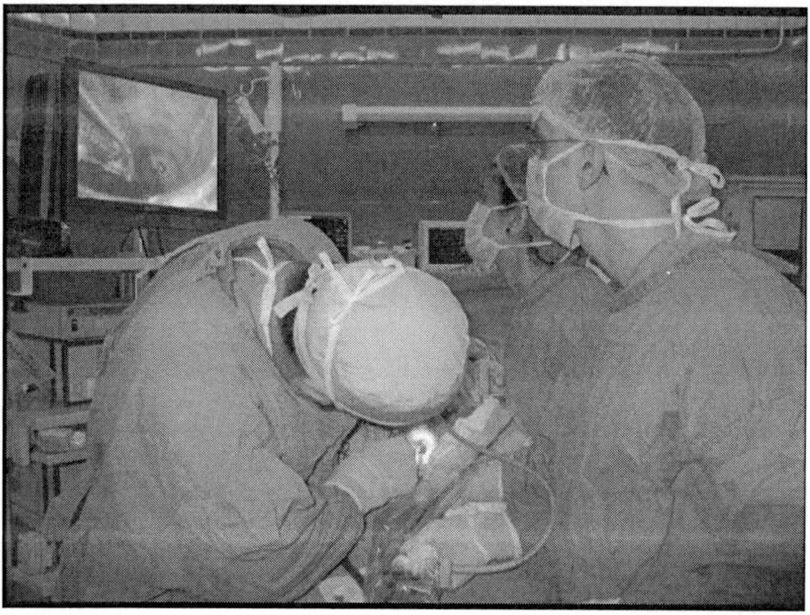

Figure 25.Surgical procedures can be watched at the monitor.

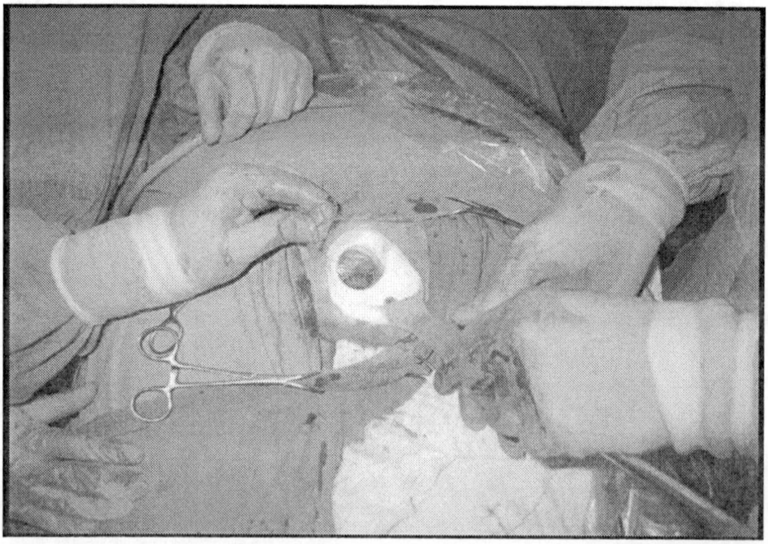

Figure 26. The front piece is taken out after the purse string suture is completed

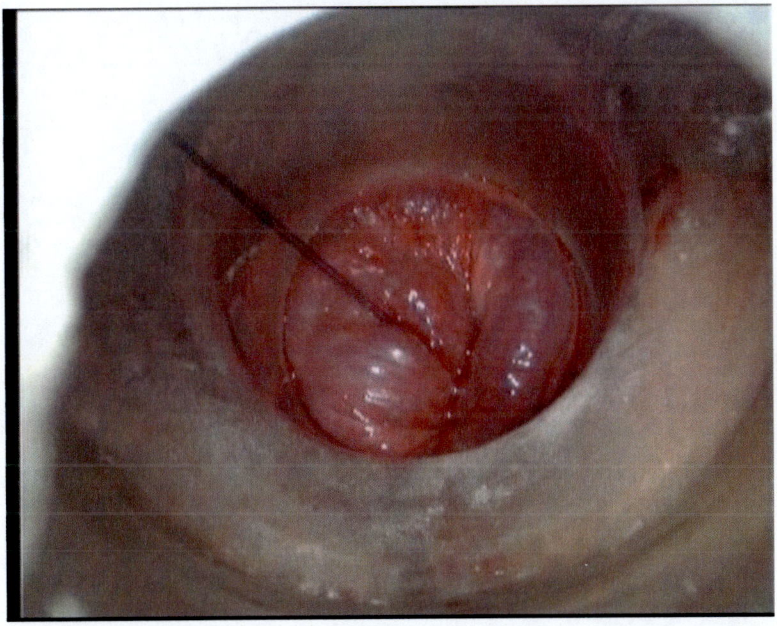

Figure 27. The purse string suture is checked after the front piece is taken out.

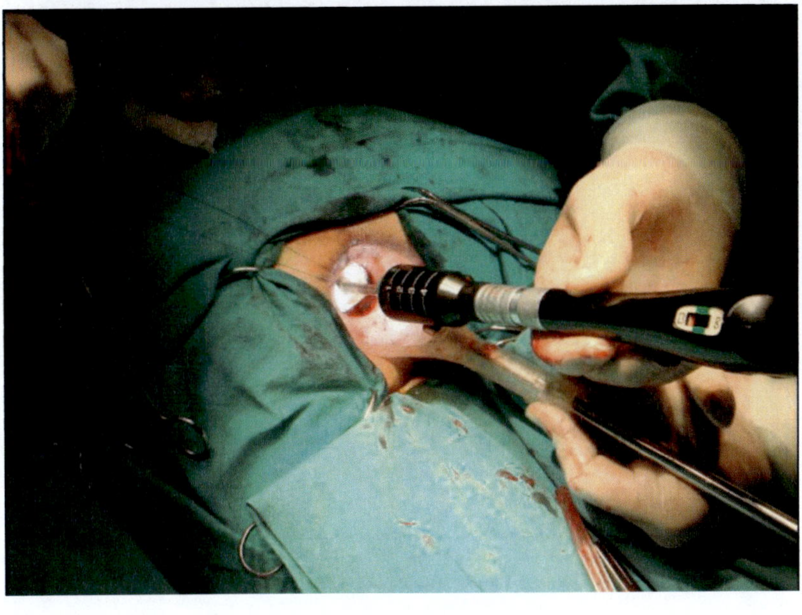

Figure 28. PPH03 stapler anvil is passed through the back piece.

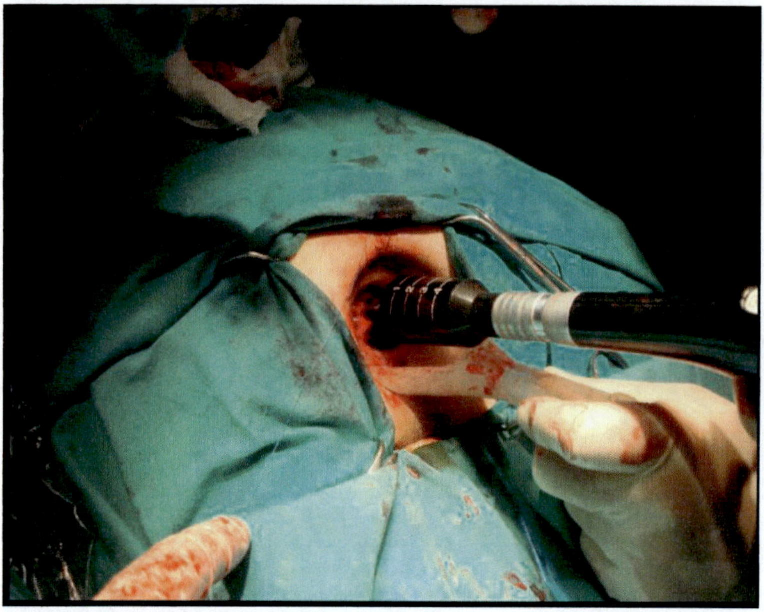

Figure 29The purse string suture is tied behind the anvil

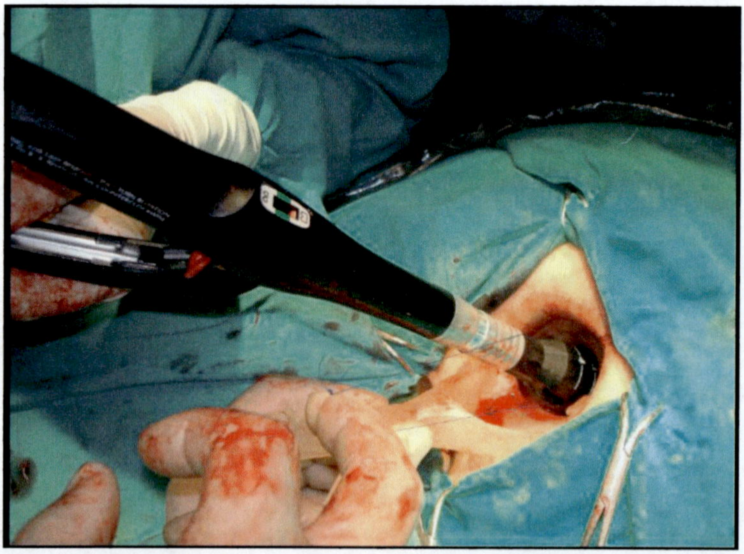

Figure 30. The stapler is fired after the hemostasis was awaited.

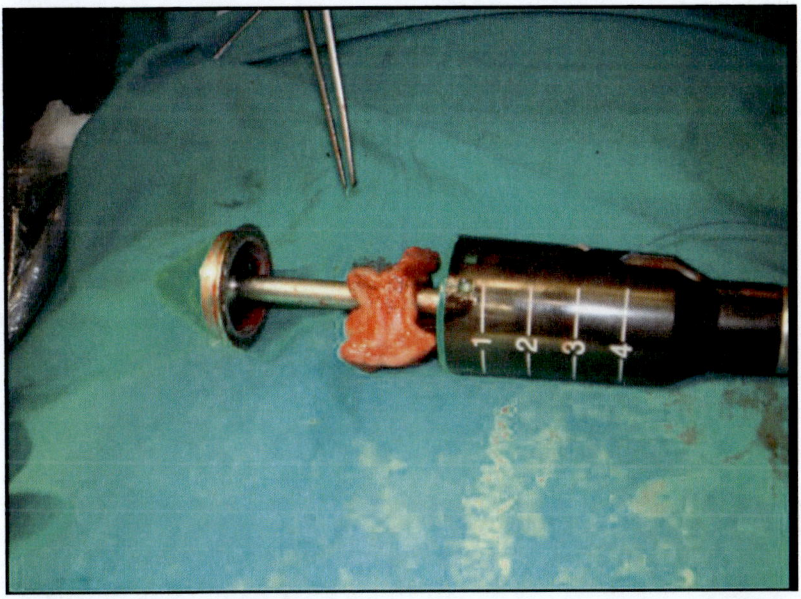

Figure 31. Ring integrity is checked.

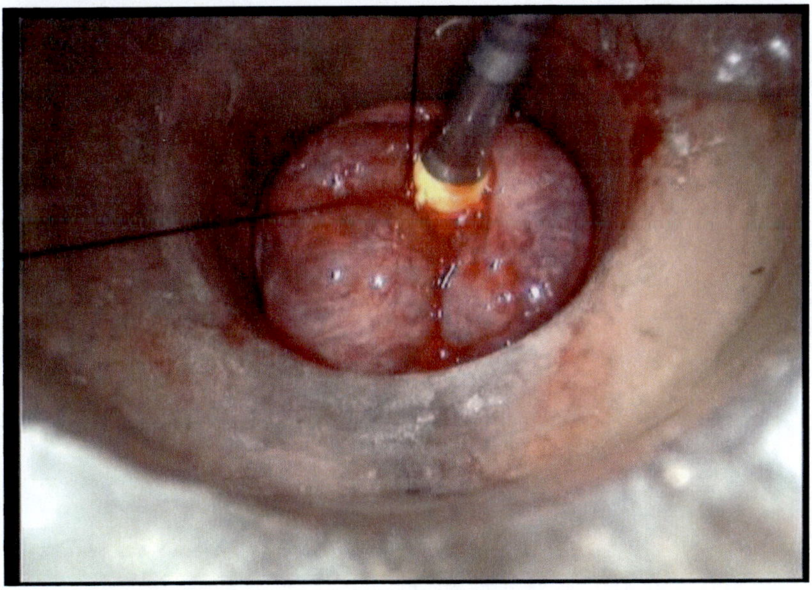

Figure 32. The purse string suture is tied by placing CEEA 34mm Stapler anvil into the rectum.

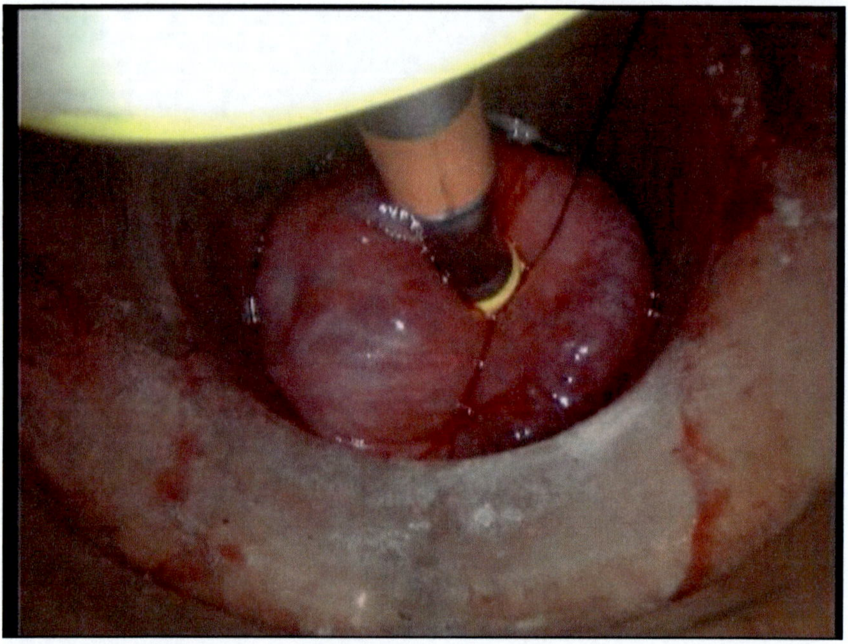

Figure 33. Anvil and stapler are combined.

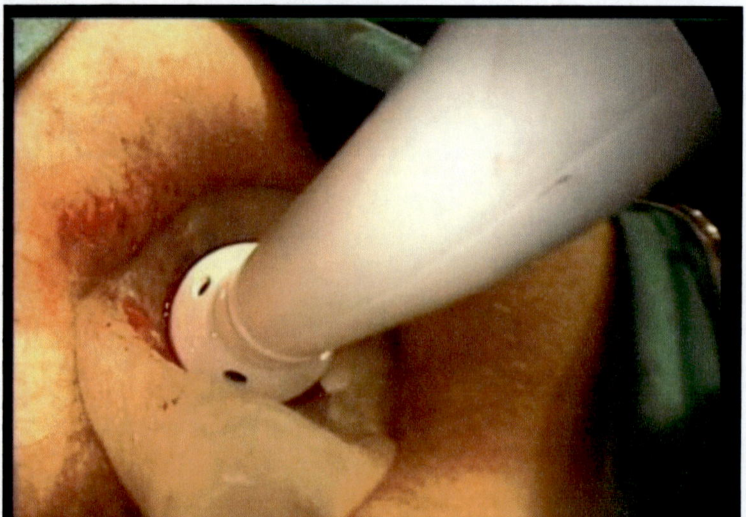

Figure 34. The stapler is fired after the hemostasis was awaited.

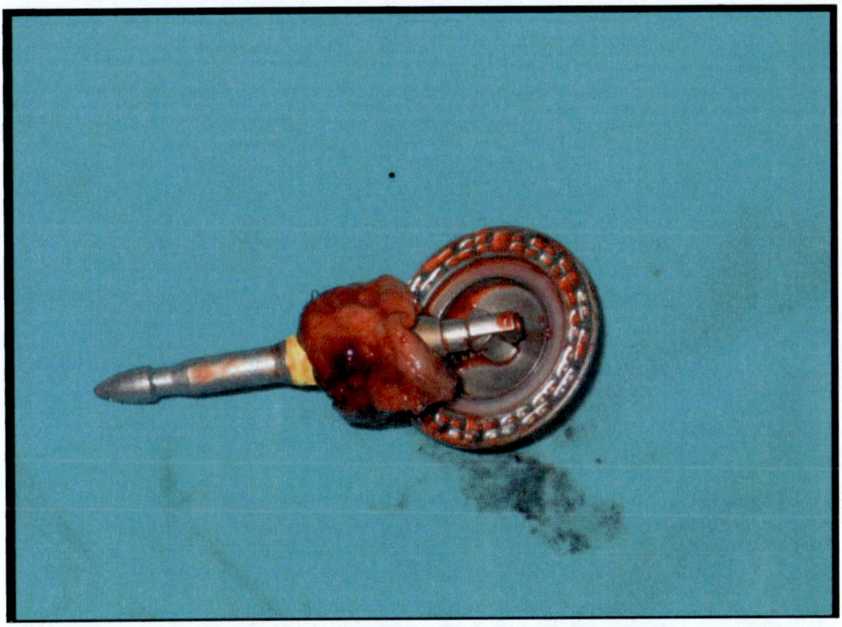

Figure 35. Ring integrity is checked.

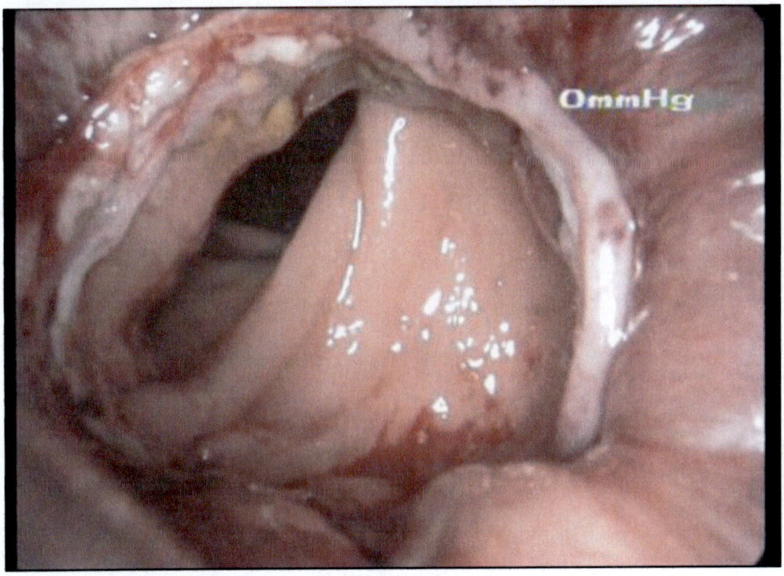

Figure 36. View of stapler line after mucosectomy.

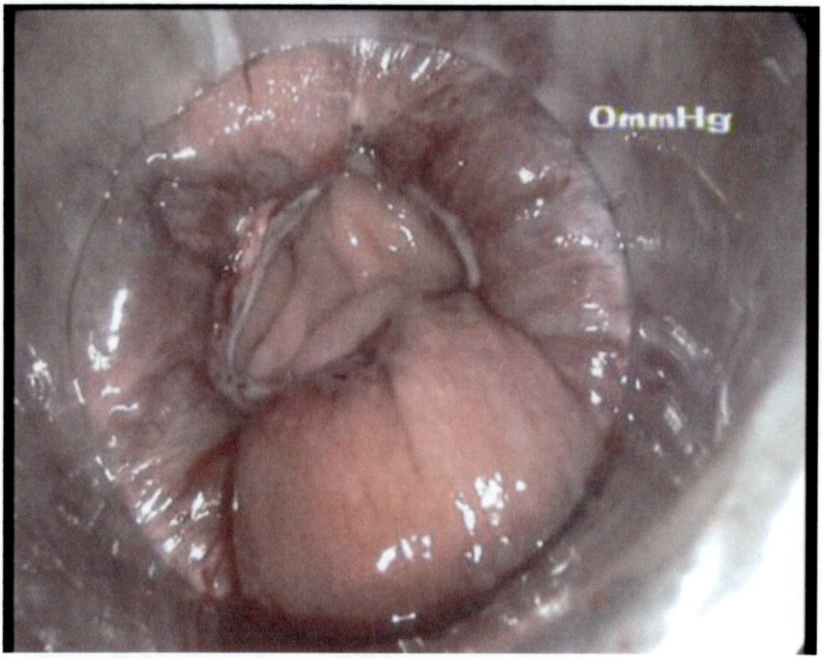

Figure 37. Stapler line is above the hemorrhoids.

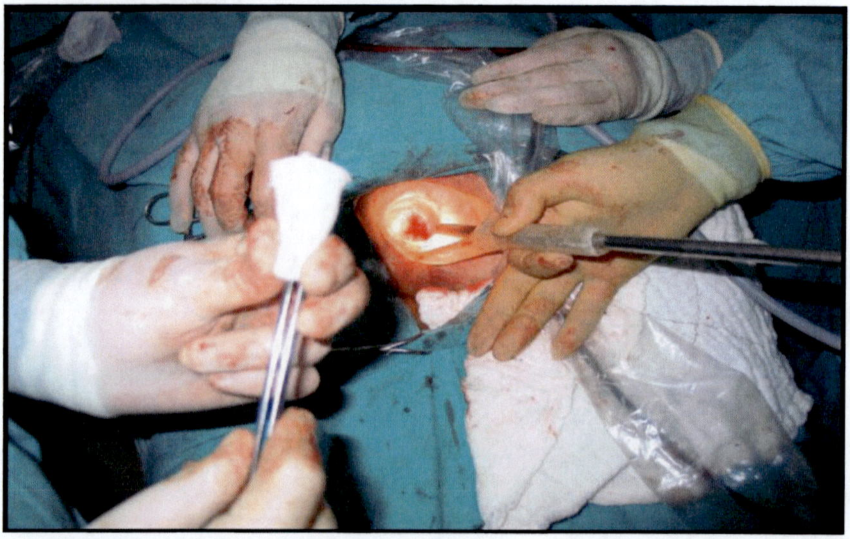

Figure 38. Spongosten is prepared.

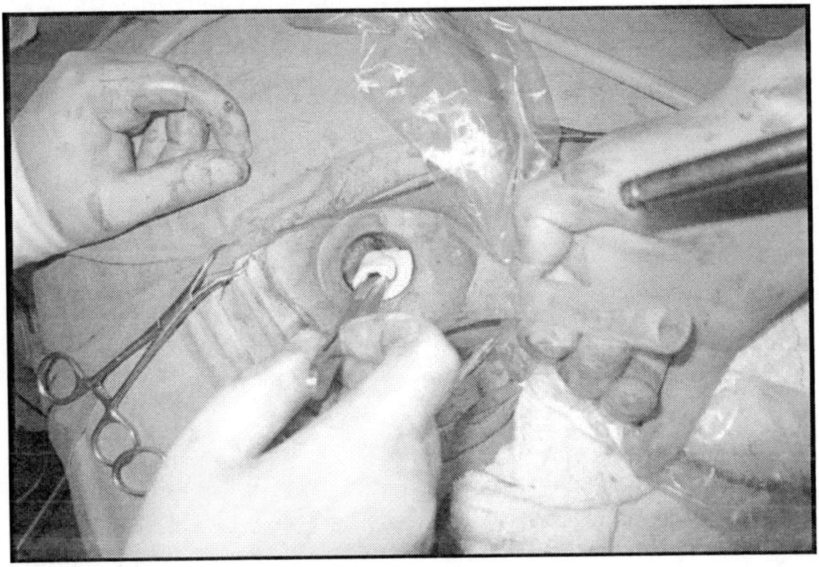

Figure 39. Spongosten is placed into the rectum after being passed through the back piece of videoanoscope.

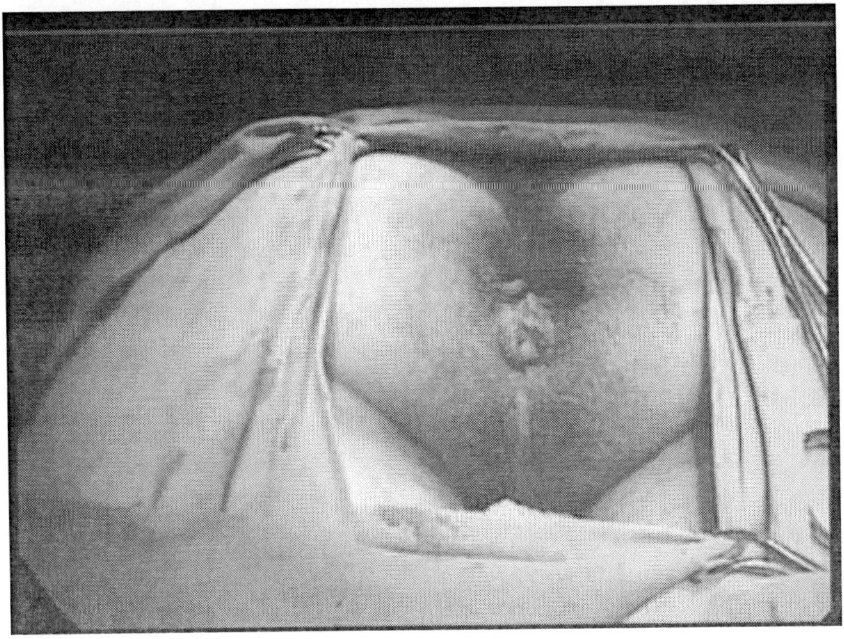

Figure 40. Postoperative view of anal region.

References

[1] Plocek MD, Kondylis LA, Duhan-Floyd N, et al. (2006) Hemorrhoidopexy staple line height predicts return to work. Dis Colon Rectum; 49:1905-1909.

[2] Bozdağ AD. A modified anoscope to facilitate the purse-string suture for stapled hemorrhoidopexy. (2005) *Tech. Coloproctol.*; 9:239-242.

[3] Bozdag AD, Nazli O, Tansug T, et al. (2007) Special anoscope for easy purse-string suture application in stapled hemorrhoidopexy. *World J. Surg.*; 31:538-541.

[4] Bozdag AD, Nazli O, Tansug T, et al. (2008) Videoanoscope assisted stapled haemorrhoidopexy: analysis of 18 patients. *Tech. Coloproctol.*; 12:123-126.

[5] Yamamoto J, Nagai M, Smith TB, et al. (2006) Adaptation of the pursestring suture anoscope with a small hole in a case of stapled hemorrhoidectomy. *Dis. Colon. Rectum.*; 49:925-926.

[6] Koh DC, Cheong DM, Wong KS. (2005) Stapled haemorrhoidectomy: bothersome staple line bleeding. *Asian J. Surg.;* 28:193-197.

[7] Jayne DG, Seow-Choen F. 2002) Modified stapled haemorrhoidopexy for the treatment of massive circumferentially prolapsing piles. *Tech. Coloproctol.*; 6:191-193.

[8] Regadas FS, Regadas SM, Rodrigues LV, et al. (2005) New devices for stapled rectal mucosectomy: a multicenter experience. *Tech. Coloproctol.;* 9:243-246.

[9] Ravo B, Amato A, Bianco V, et al. (2002) Complications after stapled hemorrhoidectomy: can they be prevented? *Tech. Coloproctol.*; 6:83-88.

[10] Tjandra JJ, Chan MKY. (2007) Systematic Review on the Procedure for Prolapse and Hemorrhoids (Stapled Hemorrhoidopexy). *Dis. Colon. Rectum.*; 50:878-892.

[11] Wong LY, Jiang JK, Chang SC, et al. (2003) Rectal perforation: a life-threatening complication of stapled hemorrhoidectomy: report of a case. *Dis. Colon. Rectum.*; 46:116-117.

[12] Aumann G, Petersen S, Pollack T, et al. (2004) Severe intra-abdominal bleeding following stapled mucosectomy due to enterocele: report of a case. *Tech. Coloproctol.*; 8:41-43.

[13] Au-Yong I, Rowsell M, Hemingway DM. (2004) Randomised controlled clinical trial of stapled haemorrhoidectomy vs conventional haemorrhoidectomy; a three and a half year follow up. *Colorectal. Dis.*; 6:37-38.

[14] Sileri P, Stolfi VM, Palimieri G, et al. (2007) Stapled hemorrhoidopexy: A popspective study from pathology to clinical outcome. *J. Gastrointes Surg.*; 11:1662-1668

[15] Rebuffat C, Porta MD, Ciccarese F, et al. (2008) A new anoscope for transanal surgery. *Am. J. Surg.*; 196:e12-e15

[16] Chew MH, Tan WS, Eu KW. (2009) The use of CEEA 34 in stapled hemorrhoidectomy: Suggested modifications in technique. *World J. Surg.*; 33: 156.

[17] Pescatori M, Quondamcarlo C. (1999) Prevention of intraoperative complications during stapled excision of rectal mucosal prolapse. *Tech. Coloproctol.*; 3:103-104.

In: Hemorrhoids: Symptoms, Diagnosis... ISBN: 978-1-60876-478-5
Authors: P. Salinitri et al., pp. 149-159

Chapter 7

NEW OPTION IN THE TREATMENT OF HEMORRHOIDAL DISEASE: DOPPLER GUIDED TRANSANAL HEMORRHOIDAL DEARTERIALISATION

Ramón Cantero
Section of Colorectal Surgery.
Hospital Infanta Sofía. Madrid (Spain)

ABSTRACT:

Hemorrhoidal disease is a common problem in the western world (in USA, ten million, just < 5 percent of the population ([1]).

Different invasive treatment modalities are available for the management of the symptomatic haemorrhoids varying from office treatment (rubber bands, sclerotherapy ,infrared coagulation, cryotherapy) and surgical procedure (hemorrhoidectomy, stapled hemorrhoidopexy)

The high frequency of this entity and the deterioration in quality of life during the initial postoperative period has led the implementation of new technique (Doppler guided transanal haemorrhoidal dearterialisation) with new devices in order to attain improved patient satisfaction (THD and haemorrhoid laser procedure).

INTRODUCTION

The prevalence of symptomatic hemorrhoids in the United States is reported to be 4,4% with a peak prevalence occurring between 45 and 65 years of age, equally in men and women.

Treatment depends on the degree of prolapse and severity of symptoms.

The existence of multiple techniques for haemorrhoidal disease demonstrates that, actually, there are no an ideal procedure.

Some of these are less aggressive[2,3] and can even be performed in the office, while others are more invasive [4,5] and require local/regional anaesthesia, and therefore an operating theatre. The first ones produce modest results and in some cases are not free from morbidity; within the second group, although long-term results are better, a higher rate of complications is found, ranging from wound infection to fecal incontinence

The choice of the best surgical technique must always be based not only on the surgeon´s personal experience but above all on the scientific evidence supporting the superiority of one surgical technique with another.

The haemorrhoidectomy is the most effective procedure for the treatment of haemorrhoidal disease [3], although not exempt from multiple potential complications and greater postoperative pain.

The last decade has showed the development of a number of minimally invasive techniques: Longo technique and doppler guided haemorrhoidal arterial ligation (DGHAL)

The mostly of the DGHAL procedures are based in the study by Morinaga in 1995 that introduced the doppler-guided haemorrhoidal dearterialisation [6]. This author, combining a proctoscopy with a doppler transducer, performed to selectively ligation of the terminal branch of the superior rectal artery (SRA) and with this the hemorrhoids´ volume is reduced which leads to an improvement in symptoms.

The doppler guided hemorrhoidal desarterialisation can be performed using a stich of coated polyglycolic acid (Transanal Haemorrhoidal Dearterialisation) or laser photocoagulation (Hemorrhoid Laser Procedure (HeLP) and Hemorrhoidoplasty).

Doppler-Guided Haemorrhoidal Arterial Ligation (Haemorrhoidal Dearterialisation)

Transanal Haemorrhoidal Dearterialisation (THD)

Transanal Haemorrhoidal Dearterialisation is one of the techniques less invasive. It utilizes a specially designed instrument, the THD.

The THD is equipped with a Doppler transducer to locate the terminal branches of the superior rectal artery, wich are then ligated, through an apposite slit in the instrument, 2-3 cm. above the dentate line (figure 1a, 1b).

Therefore, the arterial flow to the haemorrhoids is reduced and they shrink.

After ligation of the arteries, the arterial inflow to the corpus cavernosum recti (CCR) drops, the piles collapse and the eventual bleeding stops.

Once this is done, the area is tested again with the Doppler probe to ensure the absence of a distal signal in the arterial ligation.

The decreased tension allows for the regeneration of the connective tissue within the cushions. This facilitates the shrinkage of haemorrhoids and induces permanent reduction of the prolapse.

The sutures used to ligate the arteries create a rectal pexis by stitching the rectal mucosa to the layers below and elevating the haemorrhoidal cushions above the dentate line, thus reducing or eliminating the rectal prolapse (figure 2).

Nowadays, doppler guided transanal haemorrhoidal dearterialisation is considered and recommendated in grade II and III haemorrhoids [7]. DGHAL is performed as an outpatient procedure under local (with sedation), spinal or general anesthesia.

The success rate has been reported to be greater than 90% for grade III hemorrhoids [8-11], with a minimal rate of complications (mild discomfort. tenesmus, limited rectal bleeding, thrombosis). There is no anal wound to heal. There is not risk of incontinence or stricture. The failure rate is about 10 %. In a randomized study, transanal haemorrhoidal dearterialisation showed much less pain, shorter hospital stay and earlier return to work compared to hemorrhoidectomy, and long-term recurrence rates at 1 year follow-up were similar in both [12].

We have operated consecutively, *with a minimum follow-up of 3 years*, ninety patients diagnosed with grade III hemorrhoids (in press, reported preliminary study with 50 patients [13]). The indication for surgery was based on: pain-disconfort, 80(89%); bleeding, 58 (65%); prolapse, 9 (10%). The procedure was always performed under local/regional anesthesia.

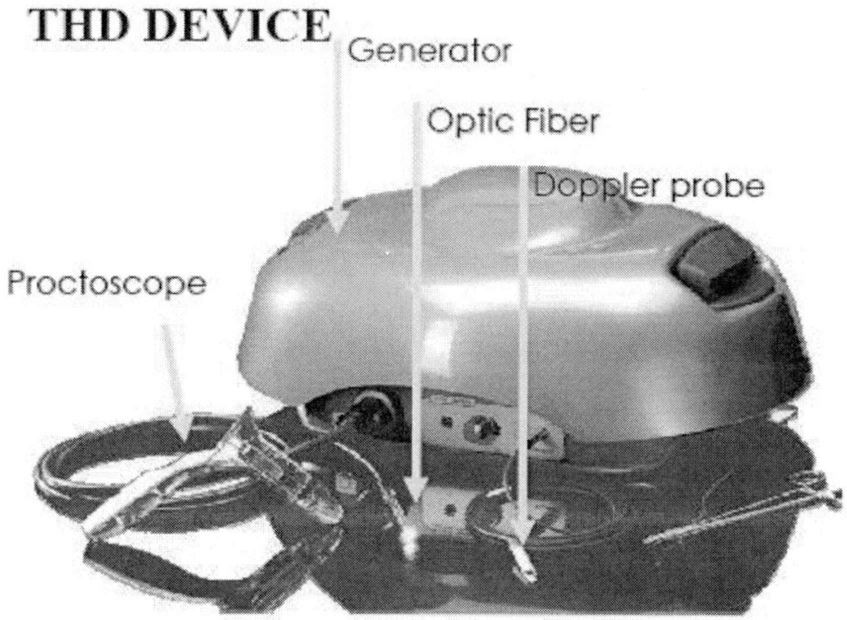

Figure 1a.- THD device.

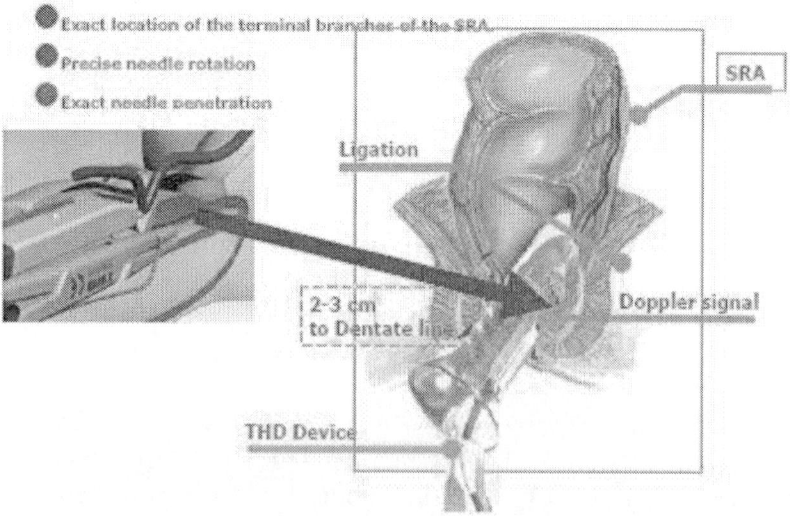

Figure 1b.- THD surgical approach.

Eight (13,7%) out of 58 patients sought medical attention for recurrent bleeding (some of them with anticoagulant chronic treatment); in three of these cases, hemorrhoidal dearterialisation was again indicated, and after the second procedure they were free of bleeding at 18, 20 and 33 months, another female patient underwent conventional hemorrhoidectomy (Milligan-Morgan technique) and another two patients were excluded from surgery since they remain asymptomatic.

Pain-disconfort was resolved in 78 patients (97,5%).

We think that doppler-guided transanal hemorrhoidal deartrialisation is a technique that must be explained to patients who are going to be operated on for hemorrhoidal disease, mentioning its advantages in terms of functional and quality of life (figure 3).

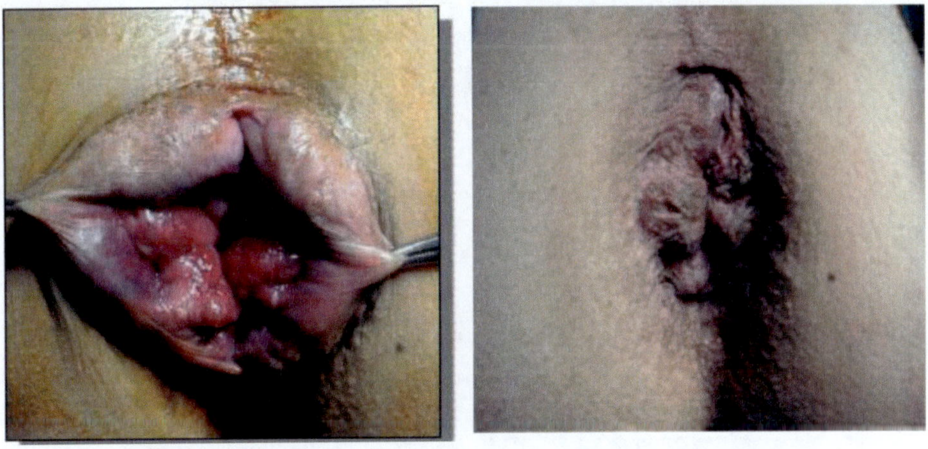

Figure 3. Clinical case. Preoperative and immediately postoperative.

HEMORRHOID LASER PROCEDURE (HELP)

A new painless outpatient technique is described for treating hemorrhoids using HeLP™ platform that is comprised of Ceralas laser 980 nm (Biolitec) with adapted proctoscope where is incorporated a high frequency doppler equipment (20 MHz)(figures 4a-4b) for fotocoagulation of the distal branches of hemorrhoidal arteries.

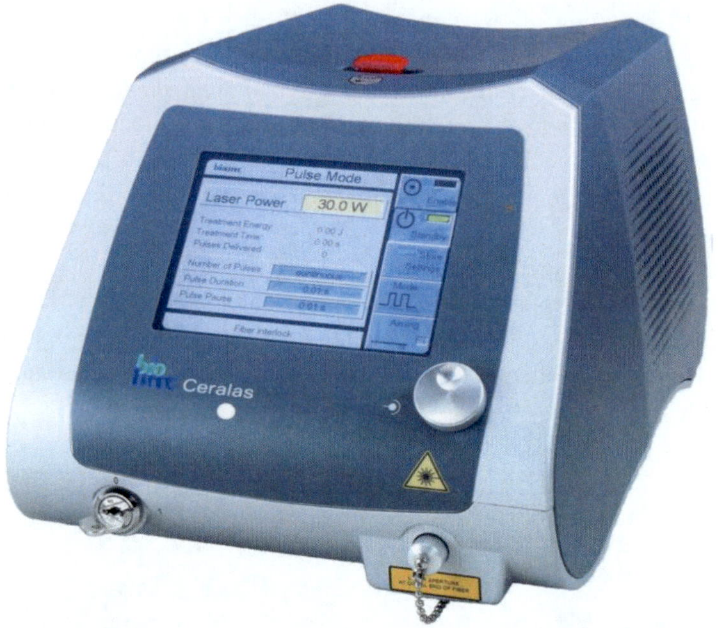

Figure 4a.- HeLP platform.

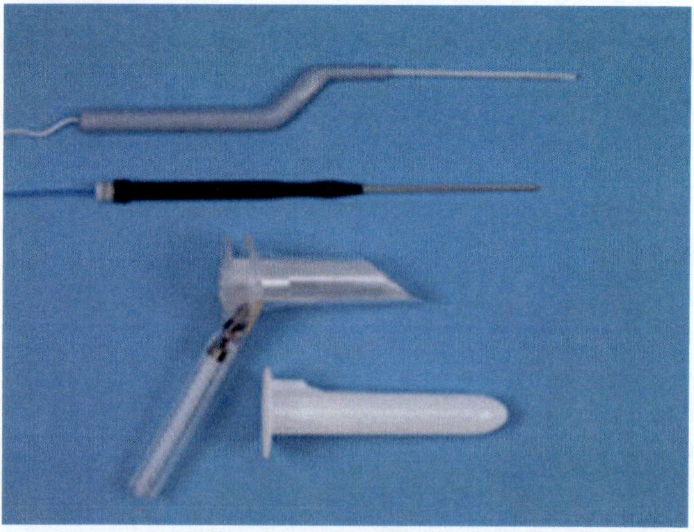

Figure 4b- Proctoscope, Doppler probe and laser fiber with handpiece.

This a new technique for treatment of hemorrhoids, based on the anatomical and aetiopathogenetic principles used for doppler-guided ligation of hemorrhoidal arteries [6], consisting of a mired fotocoagulation, with a diode laser, of the branches of the superior hemorrhoidal arteries.

The system consisted of a 980 diode laser and a set of Doppler, anoscope and light source accessory (all fornited by Biolitec, Germany) to identify and close the arteries; an aspiration probe is also provided to eliminate the fumes producted by laser coagulation of tissues.

An anoscope is inserted into the anal canal above the hemorrhoidal cushings and mired laser submucosal branches of hemorrhoidal arteries fotocoagulation, guided by ultrasound doppler (20Mhz probe of 3 mm. diameter), is done, verifying with the same doppler the arteries closure caused by laser fotocoagulation.

Fotocoagulation is done with a 1000 micron laser fibre positioned up to the rectal mucosa; coagulation is done four times with pulsed laser (each of 18 joules for a total of about 72 joules, at a potence of 14 watts) for any artery's closure.

The procedure is repeated rotating the anoscope for each of the submucosal branches of the superior hemorrhoidal arteries.

No anaesthetic or analgesic procedure is necessary.

The procedure's duration is about fifteen minutes; the treatment is ambulatory and the patient is dimitted early after operation.

More than one system was examined to facilitate the procedure and the best demonstrable was a system using a 20 Mhz laser probe encoupled with 980 laser diode and 1000 micron laser fibre, all provided by Biolitec.

Since 2002, E.Bernè have used the optical fiber and surgical laser, and included 67 patients in a study after accurate clinical evaluation and after adequate therapy. Actually for HeLP procedure we have control patients after two weeks,1 month,3 months and 8 months with good results in 2° and 3° degree hemorrhoids without severe prolapsed were not included patients with hemorrhoids of severe grade and mucosal prolapse.

Salfi and cols.[14] have reported a study with 200 patients with symptomatic second degree hemorrhoids who had episodes of anal pain, bleeding, and prolapse were treated in the past 3 years. Ambulatory treatment was done in all patients; anaesthesia or analgesia were unnecessary. Mild intraoperative and postoperative complications were seen. 91 per cent of patients have an improvement of their hemorrhoidal symptoms one to twelve months after treatment.

7, 14, 30 and 90 days (up to 12 months) after treatment the patients were examined with proctoscope.

Intraoperative complications consisted of mild pain in 10 patients (anaesthetic treatment was unnecessary), mild tenesmus in 20 patients, hemorrhagic complications that required surgical treatment (ligation) in 2 patients, bleeding requiring only laser treatment.

For 2-5 days tenesmus in 60 patients and emission of mucus or bleed in 40 patients were present ; these symptoms disappeared within 30 days in all patients without significative discomfort. .

A patient had an hemorrhagic complication at home, 7 days after treatment; he was reammitted to the hospital, but no evident hemorrhagic lesion was demonstrable endoscopically.

Doppler-guided laser treatment of hemorrhoidal arteries is, then, a good and safe method for ambulatory treatment of hemorrhoids.

Fotocoagulation causes a necrosis of rectal mucosa and submucosa and closure of arteries at doppler examination; this endoscopic necrotic aspect persists for 7-14 days after operation. Retraction of hemorrhoidal cushing are also evident after 7-14 days after operation and increase up to 90 days, determining complete or partial reduction of prolapse.

The fotocoagulation with laser of the branches of the superior hemorrhoidal arteries both close the arteries and fixs the rectal mucosa and submucosa to the muscular layer, causing a retraction of the hemorrhoids and an impediment to their prolapse through the anal canal, other than closure of the arteries.

The technique is safety and causes minimal pain or discomfort to the patient. The post operative recovery is faster than alternative approaches, with very few complications. Anaesthesia or analgesia are no longer required as it is in most other successful methods, greatly reducing complications, simplifying and making the treatment safer and faster.

The photocoagulation of terminal branches of hemorrhoidal arteries with laser system of present invention has many advantages when compared to other treatment methods. Use of small sized newly designed anoscope is relatively painless and causes less discomfort to the patient when inserted into anal opening. Since anaesthesia is not used, the patient can be discharged immediately as it is a quick and easy procedure performed in few minutes with minimal or no post-operative pain. Further with no anaesthesia required, there are no related complications.

During the procedure the position of laser fiber near to the hemorrhoidal cushion can be monitored using Doppler. This also prevents damaging of other normal vessels in the rectal and anal regions. Complete closure of each damaged artery is checked after the procedure. The sclerosis of the submucosa with fixation of the planes of the rectal wall prevents prolapse.

Patient can return to normal activity after the procedure with no or minimal post operative pain. Late and immediate results are excellent.

LASER HEMORRHOIDOPLASTY

Laser hemorrhoidoplasty (LHP) is a new painless outpatient technique described for treating III and IV grade hemorrhoids using HeLP™ platform that is comprised of Ceralas laser 980 nm (all fornited by Biolitec, Germany) with adapted proctoscope where is incorporated a high frequency doppler equipment (20 MHz)(figures 4a-4b) for fotocoagulation and It used a conic optic fiber (15 w in 3 second pulse) [15]

Laser hemorrhoidoplasty is a revolutionary development for fixed, stage four hemorrhoids. Under regional anesthesia, 1 cm long cuts are made at the less sensitive edge of the hemorrhoid nodules. After the cut is made, the nodules are scooped out from the inside with a special shaver instrument. Afterwards, they are stitched to their natural location, while the feeding artery is blocked. Additionally, the remaining arteries are found with a ultrasonic device and stitched shut.

If no contra-indications exist, an anti-inflammatory suppository placed in the rectum after the surgery. Anal tampons or other intra anal Inserts are not used, only a collecting main is placed.

After the procedure, a day-long observation of one to two-hour intervals will be done.

Due to the surgical stitches, there can be feeling of pressure for a short time. This feeling can be treated with an anti-inflammatory medicine such like diclofenac.

By means of a interstitial laser fiber, the hemorroidal knots are obliterated from the inside by application of controlled laser energy.

The mucosa and the muscle structures will be spared to a high extend, the anatomy of the rectal channel is restored and excessive arteriovenous tissue is removed and shrinked by well defined hyperthermia.

A subsequent fibrotic tissue change started which will be then removed from the body within 6 weeks. A reduction to natural tissue volume is performed without loss of tissue.

Big prolapsed knots could be fixed to their anatomical position by mucopexy. The mucosa will be lifted through vicryl ligations without generating artificial stenosis.

This treatment has the potential to improve post operative pain management due to the avoidance of open or semi-open wounds normally generated by conventional Milligan-Morgan or Ferguson techniques. The patient will experience an improved wound healing and shorter down time.

Specially in case of sequential knots this a helpful approach when use of stapler hemorrhoidopexy is not yet indicated

Long term results are not available yet.

References

[1] Bleday R, Pena JP, Rothenberg DA, Goldberg SM , Buls JG. Symptomatic hemorrhoids: current incidence and complications of operative therapy. *Dis. Colon. Rectum.* 1992;35:477-481.

[2] Ho Y-H, Tan M, Seow-Chen F. Micronized purified flavonidic fraction compared favorable with rubber band ligation and fiber alone in the management of bleeding hemorrhoids: randomized controlled trial. *Dis. Colon. Rectum.* 2000; 43:66-9.

[3] Mc Rae HM, Mc Leod RS. Comparison of hemorrhoidal treatment modalities: a meta-analysis. *Dis. Colon. Rectum.* 1995; 38: 687-694

[4] Oh C. Problems of cryohemorrhoidectomy. *Cryobiology* 1982; 19: 283-6

[5] Longo A. Treatment oh hemorrhoidal disease by reduction of mucosa and hemorrhoidal prolapse with circular stapling device: a new procedure. 6th World Congress of Endoscopic Surgery. Bologna: Monduzzi Editore, 1998: 777-84

[6] Morinaga K, Hasuda K, Ikeda T. A novel therapy for internal hemorrhoids: ligation of the hemorrhoidal artery with a newly devised instrument (moricorn) in conjunction with a doppler flowmeter. *Am. J. Gastroenterology* 1995; 90: 610-13

[7] Altomare DF, Roveran A, Pecorella G, Gaj F, Stortini E. The treatment of haemorrhoids. Guidelines of the Italian Society of Colorectal Surgery. (www.SICCR.org).

[8] Sohn N, Aronoff JS, Cohen FS, Weinstein MA. Transanal hemorrhoidal dearterialisation is an alternative to operative hemorrhoidectomy. *Am. J. Surg.* 2001; 182: 515-19.

[9] Ramirez JM, Aguilella V, Elia M et al. Doppler-guided hemorrhoidal artery ligation in the management of symptomatic hemorrhoids. *Rev. Esp. Enferm. Dig.* 2005; 97: 97-103.

[10] Felice G, Privitera A, Ellul E, Klaumann M. Doppler-guided hemorrhoidal artery ligation. An alternative to hemorrhoidectomy. *Dis. Colon. Rectum.* 2005; 48: 2090-2093.

[11] Greenberg R, Karin E, Avital S et al. First 100 cases with doppler-guided hemorrhoidal artery ligation. *Dis. Colon. Rectum.* 2006; 485-9.

[12] Bursics A, Morvay K, Kupcsulik P, Flautner L. Comparison of early and 1 year follow-up results of conventional hemorrhoidectomy and haemorrhoid artery ligation: a randomized study. *Int. J. Colorectal Dis.* 2004; 19: 176-180

[13] Cantero R, Balibrea JM, Ferrigni C, Sanz M, García Pérez JC, Pérez R, Luffiego A, Balibrea JL. Desarterialización hemorroidal transanal guiada por Doppler. Una alternativa en el tratamiento de las hemorroides. *Cir .Esp.* 2008;83(5):248-51.

[14] Salfi R. A new technique for ambulatory hemorrhoidal treatment. Doppler-guided laser photocoagulation of hemorrhoidal arteries. *Coloproctology* 2009; 31:99-103.

[15] Karahaliloˇglu AF. Erste Ergebnisse der Laserobliteration von erst- bis zweitgradigen Hämorrhoiden. *Coloproctology* 2007;29:327–36.

In: Hemorrhoids: Symptoms, Diagnosis… ISBN: 978-1-60876-478-5
Authors: P. Salinitri et al., pp. 161- 171

Chapter 8

ANAL ULTRA SLOW WAVE: A MYSTERIOUS MANOMETRIC FINDING WITH HEMORRHOIDS

***Hiroyuki Kayaba*[1]**

Department of Infection, Allergy, Clinical Immunology and Laboratory Medicine, Akita University Graduate School of Medicine, Japan

ABSTRACT

Anal ultra slow wave (USW) is a manometric finding observed in some patients with hemorrhoids and is assumed to represent a hyperactive internal anal sphincter. Lateral sphincterotomy has been reported as a treatment option in patients with hemorrhoids exhibiting USW to reduce the activity of the internal anal sphincter. Hemorrhoids in the anal canal were once thought to induce USW; however, the underlining mechanism of USW is not known. Hyperactivity of the internal anal sphincter, namely hypertonic anal canal, may cause difficulty in defecation. In fact, USW is also observed in some patients without hemorrhoids but with megacolon, chronic constipation, spina bifida, and anal fissure. We found USW in four out of 70 children with chronic constipation. The origin of USW is thought to be the internal anal sphincter because some patients with spina bifida with a completely flaccid external anal sphincter can exhibit USW. The natural history of patients with USW is not known. In some cases, histological change in intestinal ganglion cells is observed. In this commentary, USW is presented and its clinical

---

1 Hondo, Akita 010-8543, Japan ,Phone and FAX: +88-18-884-6248, e-mail:kayaba@hos.akita-u.ac.jp.

relevance is discussed with a special interest to the manometric findings of hemorrhoids.

I. Introduction

Anatomically, the term "hemorrhoids" refers to cushions of tissue filled with blood vessels at the junction of the rectum and anus, while surgically it refers to varicosities of hemorrhoid tissue, or hyperplasia of the corpus cavernosum recti [1], a common surgical condition of the anus. Surgical treatment for hemorrhoids is well established and widely accepted; however, the physiopathology still remains to be clarified. Since hemorrhoids are a varicosity, conditions that increase venous pressure such as increased straining during bowel movements, pregnancy and portal hypertension may cause hemorrhoids. It is acceptable that such conditions that increase venous pressure may cause hemorrhoids, whereas the reason why patients with hemorrhoids tend to experience increased straining during bowel movements needs further discussion. Very slow rhythmic pressure fluctuation with a frequency of 0.5 – 2/min has been observed in manometric studies of the anus in some populations with hemorrhoids. This very slow rhythmic activity is called ultra slow wave (USW). USW is seen not only in patients with hemorrhoids but also in several other clinical conditions. In this commentary, USW and its clinical relevance are discussed.

II. Manometric Findings Associated with Hemorrhoids

1. High Anal Resting Pressure

Reports of at least 15 studies have been published since Hancock et al. (1975) [2] reported high anal resting pressure in subjects with hemorrhoids (Table 1). All but one of these studies reported a statistically significant higher maximal anal resting pressure in subjects with hemorrhoids as compared with controls with; however, the method of measurement differed in each study. The ratio of maximal anal resting pressure in subjects with hemorrhoids to that in controls calculated based on these studies was an average of 1.29±0.16 and ranged from in 0.94 to 1.54.

Table 1 Comparison of maximal anal resting pressure between hemorrhoid patients and control

Author (year)	Method	Hemorrhoid		Control		Patients/Control ratio
		Mean maximal anal resting pressure (H_2O)	n	Mean maximal anal resting pressure (H_2O)	n	
Hancock BD et al. (1975) [2)]	Balloon	93,6	56	66,8	40	1,40
Hancock BD (1976) [3)]	Balloon	107,8	50	85	50	1,27
Arabi Y et al. (1977) [4)]	Balloon	106	119	88	31	1,21
Creve U et al. (1979) [5)]	Balloon	99,8	28	94,7	32	1,05
Hiltunen KM et al. (1985) [6)]	Perfused open tip	106	38	96	29	1,10
El-Gendi MA-F et al. (1986) [7)]	Perfused open tip	109	30	88	20	1,24
Schouten WR et al. (1986) [8)]	Microtransducer	152	84	109	40	1,39
Deutch AA et al. (1987) [9)]	Balloon	139	18	104	19	1,34
Roe AM et al. (1987) [10)]	Balloon	128,3	50	84,5	36	1,52
Lin JK (1989) [11)]	Perfused opent p	116	145	96,8	78	1,20
Champigneulle B et al. (1989) [12)]	Perfused open tip	136	22	98	33	1,39

Table 1. (Continued)

Author (year)	Method	Hemorrhoid		Control		Patients/Control ratio
		Mean maximal anal resting pressure (H_2O)	n	Mean maximal anal resting pressure (H_2O)	n	
Schouten WR et al. (1992)[13)]	Microtransducer	154	20	112	20	1,38
Sun WM et al. (1992)[14)]	Balloon	62	25	45	22	1,38
Faurouk R et al. (1994)[15)]	Microtransducer	116*	16	94*	20	1,23
Eckardt V et al. (1997)[16)]	Perfused open tip	59*	58	63*	20	0,94
Chauhan A et al. (2007)[17)]	Perfused open tip	69.4*	25	45.2*	25	1,54

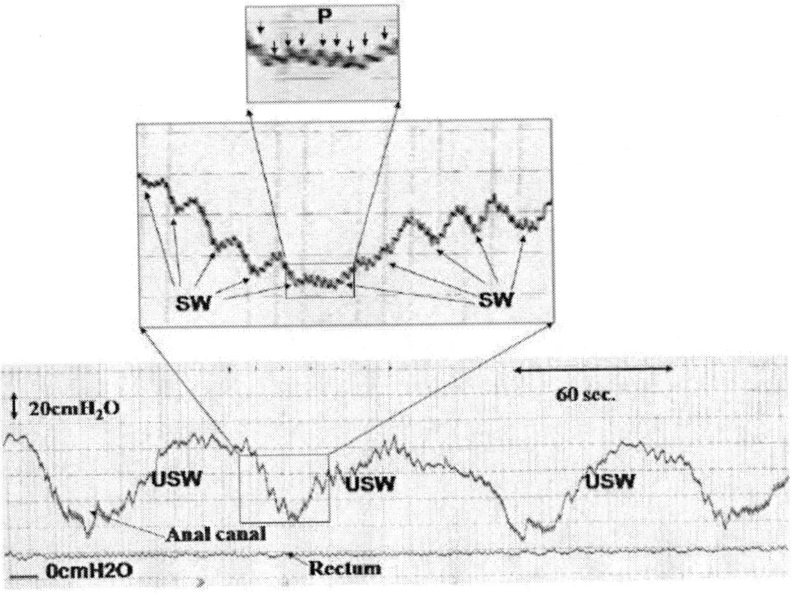

Figure 1. Pressure fluctuations of the anal canal. Three kinds of pressure fluctuations are presented, namely, small pulsating waves (p) reflecting vascular pressure, slow waves (SW) with a frequency of 10 – 20/min and ultraslow waves (USW).

2. Ultra Slow Waves of the Anal Canal

There are three kinds of pressure fluctuations in the anal canal, i.e., small pulsating waves reflecting vascular pressure, slow waves with a frequency of 10 – 20/min and USW (Figure 1). Ultra slow waves are rhythmical pressure fluctuations with a frequency less than 2/min and an amplitude greater than 25 cm H_2O [3]. It is recommended that the physician make sure that these giant waves are lacking synchronicity with rectal contractions and that they have persistent slow waves at their nadir [20] because repeated recto-anal inhibitory reflex caused by rectal contractions resembles USW in shape. The prevalence rate of USW in patients with hemorrhoids has been reported in more than 10 reports to date (Table 2). The prevalence rate of USW in these reports varies with a range of 8 – 100% in patients and 0 – 10% in controls. In total, 125 of 323 (38.7%) patients with hemorrhoids and 17 of 345 (4.9%) controls were positive for USW. Furthermore, anal pressure in subjects with USW was significantly higher than that in subjects without USW [2, 9, 13, 16, 19, 20].

Table 2 Prevalence of USW

Reference	Method	USW			
		Subjects with hemorrhoids		Controls	
		Positive/Total	%	Positive/Total	%
Hancock BD et al. (1975) [2]	Balloon	22/56	39,0	3/40	7,5
Hancock BD (1976) [3]	Balloon	17/40	42,0	4/84	5,0
Read MG et al. (1982) [18]	Perfused open tip	7/24	29,2	NA	NA
El-Gendi MA-F et al. (1986) [7]	Perfused open tip	4/30	13,3	0/20	0,0
Roe AM et al. (1987) [10]	Balloon	16/40	40,0	0/19	0,0
Champigneulle B et al. (1989) [12]	Perfused open tip	15/25	60,0	2/22	9,1
Schouten WR et al. (1992) [13]	Microtransducer	29/58	50,0	2/20	10,0
Faurouk R et al. (1994) [15]	Microtransducer	10/22	45,5	2/33	6,1
Eckardt V et al. (1997) [16]	Perfused open tip	2/25	8,0	0/25	0,0
Yoshino H et al. (2007) [19]	Perfused open tip	NA	NA	0/32	0,0
Yoshino H et al. (2007) [20]	Perfused open tip	3/3	100,0	4/50	4,1
	Total	125/323	38,7	17/345	4,9

That is why USWs are thought to represent hyperactivity of the internal anal sphincter. Induction of anesthesia or complete paralysis of the external anal sphincter has no effect on USW [21], while lateral internal sphincterotomy or forced dilatation of the anal canal may cause disappearance of USW [2, 13]. The underlying mechanism of UWS and high anal pressure has yet to be elucidated. The hypothesis that peristaltic activity of the internal anal sphincter generates USW [10] does not explain the emergence of UWS in several other conditions such as chronic constipation and megacolon[20)] and in normal subjects.

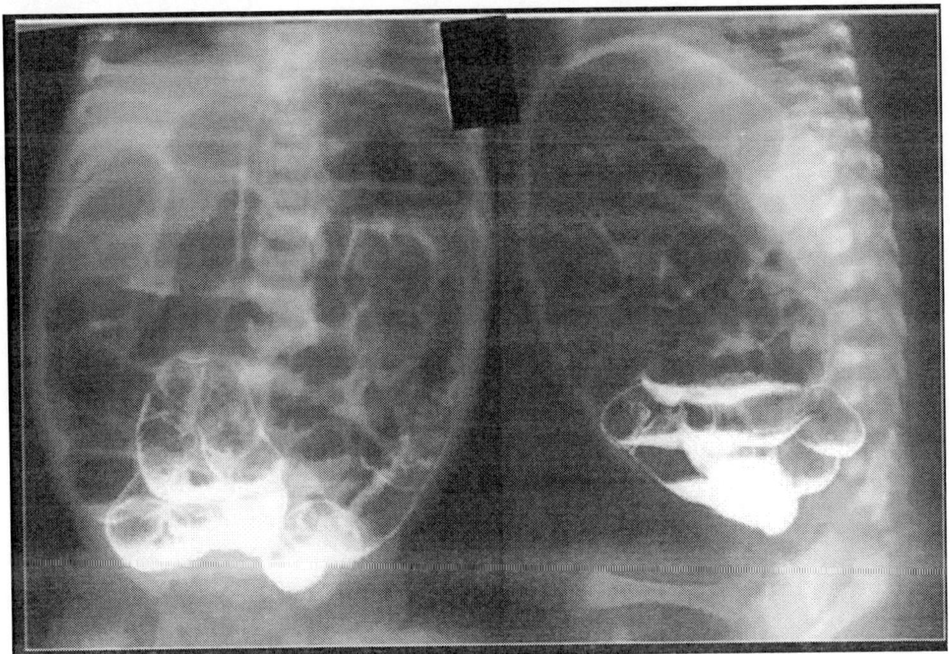

Figure 2. Abdominal X-ray films of an infant with USWs.
Marked intestinal gas and the remnant of contrast enema is seen. (lt: supine position, A-P view, rt: upright-lateral view).

III. USW-Related Clinical Conditions

Ultra slow wave of the anal canal is not a specific manometric finding for hemorrhoids. Since USW accompanies hyperactivity of the internal anal sphincter and high anal pressure, patients with USW tend to share a common problem, namely, difficulty in defecation. Excessive straining at stool is a frequent complaint of these patients. Fecoflowmetric evaluation of the ability to pass stool in these patients showed intermittent excretion from the rectum with a low flow rate and long excretion time [19]. During the early infantile period, they exhibit marked abdominal distension (Figure 2), vomiting, and constipation, mimicking Hirschsprung's disease. It is not uncommon for patients with UWS to fail to show typical recto-anal inhibitory reflex, which makes exclusion of Hirschsprung's disease difficult with a manometric study. In addition to chronic constipation and hemorrhoids, megacolon was a typical clinical presentation in our adult cases. Some of these patients had undergone surgery for dilated colonic loop with unsatisfactory long-term results before their first visit to our clinic [20]. Furthermore, a high incidence of accompanying neurological disorders may warrant attention. In our adult series [20], three of 10 patients with USW had concomitant central nervous system disorders, and of four pediatric cases, one girl with severe chronic constipation developed epilepsy at the age of 10 years, two years after her first visit [19]. Disappearance of USW during sleep [15] may suggest the influence of the central nervous system on development of USW.

4. Natural History of Patients with USW

No study has ever published on the natural history of patients with USW because our report published in 2007 [19] was the first in pediatric cases, and the follow-up period is still too short. At least in infantile cases, symptoms are well controlled with conservative treatment such as laxatives and temporal use of suppository or glycerin enema. There is little information available to answer whether or not these pediatric cases will become adult patients with chronic constipation, hemorrhoids and/or megacolon in the future.

5. Pathological Findings

Of our 14 cases, pathological examination was carried out in two pediatric cases in their infantile period and one adult case. Suction biopsy of the rectal wall in one infant revealed increased acetylcholinesterase activity and ganglion cells, while there was no abnormality was noted ininfant. A 74-year-old woman with megacolon and chronic constipation, who lacked recto-anal inhibitory reflex, had hyperplastic ganglion cells in her rectal wall (Figure 3).

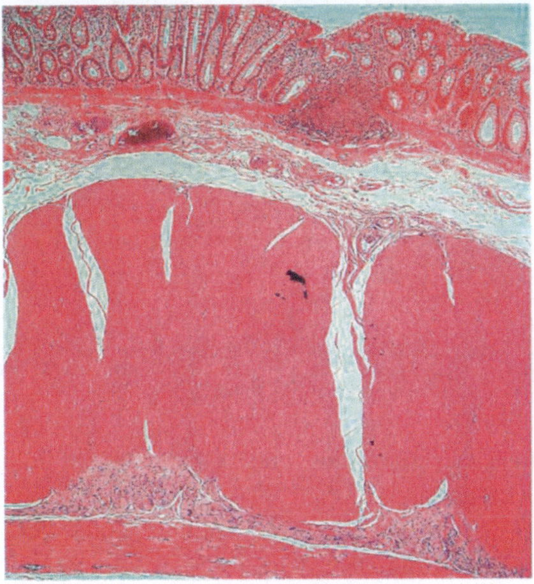

Figure 3.

6. Treatment

To relieve hyperactivity of the internal anal sphincter, lateral internal sphincterotomy or forceful dilatation of the anal canal is proposed as surgical treatment [2, 5, 22]. Since glyceryl trinitrate, acting as an NO donor, decreases internal anal sphincter tone with disappearance of USW [23], topical use of glyceryl trinitrate ointment is proposed as the medical treatment of choice in recent years [24, 25].

7. Conclusion

USW is a manometric finding frequently seen in patients with hemorrhoids; however, it is not specific to hemorrhoids. USW represents hyperactivity of the internal anal sphincter and, as a result, may be seen in several conditions caused by tonic internal anal sphincter. As was shown in this commentary, USW-presenting conditions such as chronic constipation, hemorrhoids, and megacolon in adults and marked abdominal distension mimicking **Hirschsprung's disease** in infants may share a common physiopathology; however, there remain questions to be investigated.

ACKNOWLEDGEMENTS

Our works on USW were supported by the Mitsubishi Foundation Research Grants and Assocation for Technical Aids Research Grants.

REFERENCES

[1] Loder PB et a.l., Haemorrhoids: pathology, pathophysiology and aetiology, *Br. J. Surg.* 81:946-954, 1994
[2] Hancock BD et al., The internal sphincter and **Lord's procedure for** haemorrhoids Br J Surg 62:833-836, 1975
[3] Hancock BD, Measurement of anal pressure and motility, *Gut* 17:645-651, 1976.
[4] Arabi Y et a。 l, Anal pressures in hemorrhoids and anal fissure *Am. J. Surg. 134:608-610, 1977.*
[5] Creve U et a。 l, **The effect of Lord's procedure on anal pressure**, *Dis. Colon. Rectum.* 22:483-485, 1979
[6] Hiltunen KM et al., Anal manometric findings in symptomatic hemorrhoids, *Dis. Colon. Rectum.*28:807-809, 1985
[7] El-Gendi MA-F et al., Anorectal pressure in patients with symptomatic hemorrhoids, *Dis .Clon. Rectum.* 29:388-391, 1986
[8] Schouten WR et al., Lateral internal sphincterotomy in the treatment of hemorrhoids. A clinical and manometric study.*Dis. Colon. Rectum*. 29:869-872, 1986
[9] Deutch AA et al., Anal pressure measurements in the study of hemorrhoid etiology and their relation to treatment, *Dis. Colon. Rectum* 30:855-857, 1987
[10] Roe AM et al., Submucosal versus ligation excision haemorrhoidectomy: a comparison of anal sensation, anal sphincter manometry and postoperative pain and function, *Br. J. Surg* .74:948-951, 1987
[11] Lin JK, Anal manometric studies in hemorrhoids and anal fissures, *Dis Colon. Rectum. 3*2:839-842, 1989

[12] Champigneulle B et al.,Effect of hemorrhoidectomy on anal sphincterfunction: a prospective study, *Gastroenterol. Clin. Biol.* 13:452-456, 1989
[13] Schouten WR et al, Ultra slow wave pressure variations in the anal canal before and after lateral internal sphincterotomy, *Int. J. Colorect. Dis*. 7:115-118, 1992
[14] Sun WM et al., Haemorrhoids are associated not with hypertrophy of the internal anal sphincter, but with hypertension of the anal cushions, *Br. J. Surg.* 79:592-594, 1992
[15] Faurouk R et al., Sustained internal sphincter hypertonia in patients with chronic anal fissure, *Dis. Colon. Rectum* .37:424-429, 1994
[16] Eckardt V et al., Anal ultra slow waves- a smooth muscle phenomenon associated with dyschezia, *Dig. Dis. Sci.* 42:2439-2445, 1997
[17] Chauhan A et al., Randomized controlled trial to assess the role of raised anal pressures in the pathogenesis of symptomatic early hemorrhoids, *Dig. Surg.* 24:28-32, 2007
[18] Read MG et al., A prospective study of the effect of haemorrhoidectomy on sphincter function and faecal continence, *Br. J. Surg* .69:396-398, 1982
[19] Yoshino H et al., Anal ultraslow waves and high anal pressure in childhood: a clinical condition mimicking Hirschsprung disease, *J. Pediatr. Surg.*, 42:1422-1428, 2007
[20] Yoshino H et al., Megacolon hemorrhoids and constipation: multiple clinical presentations of anal ultra slow waves and high anal pressure, Tohoku *J. Exp. Med.*, 211: 127-132, 2007
[21] Wankling WJ et al., Basal electrical activity in the anal canal in man, *Gut,*9:457-460, 1968
[22] Shouten WR et al., Lateral internal sphincterotomy in the treatment of hemorrhoids, *Dis. Colon. Rectum.* 29:869-872, 1986
[23] Bassotti G et al., Double-blind manometric assessment of two topical glyceryl trinitrate formulations in patients with chronic anal fissures, *Digest. Liver Dis.* 32:699-702, 2000
[24] Bhardwaj R, Neuromyogenic properties of the internal anal sphincter: therapeutic rationale for anal fissures, *Gut* 46:861-868, 2000
[25] Tjandra JJ et al., Rectogesic® (glyceryl trinitrate 0.2%) ointment relieves symptoms of haemorrhoids associated with high resting anal canal pressures, *Colorectal Dis.*9:457-463, 2006

INDEX

B

C

D

E

F

G

H

I

J

K

L

M

N

O

P

Q

R

T

U

V

W